Illustrated Hairdressing Dictionary

Jane Hiscock
Nicci Moorman
Leah Palmer

www.heinemann.co.uk

✓ Free online support
✓ Useful weblinks
✓ 24 hour online ordering

01865 888118

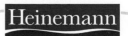

Heinemann is an imprint of Pearson Education Limited, a company incorporated in England and Wales, having its registered office at Edinburgh Gate, Harlow, Essex, CM20 2JE. Registered company number: 872828

www.heinemann.co.uk

Heinemann is a registered trademark of Pearson Education Limited

Text © Jane Hiscock, Nicci Moorman, Leah Palmer 2008

First published 2008

12 11 10 09 08
10 9 8 7 6 5 4 3 2

British Library Cataloguing in Publication Data is available from the British Library on request.

ISBN 978 0 435464 89 9

43540t
646.724094
(Reference)

Edited by Mary Mackill
Typeset by Saxon Graphics Limited
Original illustrations © Pearson Education Limited 2008
Picture research by Susi Paz
Cover photo © Jupiter Images
Printed in China (CTPS/02)

Websites
The websites used in this book were correct and up to date at the time of publication. It is essential for tutors to preview each website before using it in class so as to ensure that the URL is still accurate, relevant and appropriate. We suggest that tutors bookmark useful websites and consider enabling students to access them through the school/college intranet.

Contents

Acknowledgements

The authors and publisher would like to thank the following individuals and organisations for permission to reproduce copyright material.

Photo Acknowledgements
Page 2 – © Bella Hair; pages 4, 162 (a) and (c), 163 (a) – © Medical-on-Line/Alamy; pages 7, 11, 12, 14, 19, 20, 23 (b), 25, 30, 33, 34, 37, 38, 43, 52, 64, 65, 66 (a), 70, 75, 79, 84, 88, 91, 95, 99, 102, 103, 106, 107, 113, 119, 120, 121, 123, 124, 129, 130, 134, 135, 138, 142, 144, 149, 154 – © Pearson Education Ltd./Gareth Boden; page 9 – © Goldwell; page 23 (a) – © WAHL; page 44 – © John Carne; page 49 – © Bubbles Photolibrary/Alamy; pages 50, 77, 146 – © Pearson Education Ltd./Chris Honeywell; page 62 – © Dr Chris Hale/Science Photo Library; page 66 (b) – © iStockPhotos/Kamil Karpiel; pages 162 (b), 163 (b) – © St Bartholomew's Hospital/Science Photo Library; page 163 (c) – © Custom Medical Stock Photo/Alamy.

Authors' Acknowledgements
Jane Hiscock dedicates her contribution to Stephen, her husband, who took over the domestics while she was locked in combat with the computer, and Victoria and Venetia, her beauty therapist daughters, with love and thanks.

Nicci Moorman would like to thank her husband, Mark, and daughter, Jessica, for their patience and understanding and the hours they spent entertaining each other to enable her to work on her contribution.

Leah Palmer is grateful for the patience and forbearance of her family: Kev, Brandon and Phoebe. Without their unconditional love and support she would not have juggled a full-time job, met deadlines and kept her sanity!

All three authors would like to record how much they've enjoyed working with each other on this dictionary, and with Heinemann's in-house team.

Introduction

Welcome to your Illustrated Hairdressing Dictionary; a uniquely useful reference book which we hope will serve you well whether you are studying towards a Hairdressing qualification or starting out in the Hairdressing and Barbering profession.

We understand the many uses of an at-a-glance guide; whether you use it as part of your revision, for additional support after lessons; when preparing work during your personal study time or to refresh your knowledge in the salon.

In compiling this dictionary, our aim was to provide an easy-to-follow guide to the many technical and professional words you'll encounter in the constantly-updating world of Hairdressing and Barbering. We've also included words that you may encounter as part of your assessments and assignments so you can be clear about what is expected of you. Each entry has a clear and simple definition and pronunciation guide, with a more detailed explanation where necessary, and we've added plenty of illustrations where they are most useful – sometimes a picture really is worth a thousand words!

This dictionary is based on key terms and phrases from the National Occupational Standards (NOS) for Hairdressing, Levels 1 to 3, and includes the following information:

- Common terms used during the assessment process to help you understand what is being asked of you
- Technical terms you will encounter in the classroom or when carrying out practical treatments

Introduction

- Professional terms that you will encounter in the hairdressing industry
- An illustrated appendix to provide easy access to some of the more challenging areas such as:
    - underpinning anatomy and physiology to put individual terms in context
    - an overview of relevant legislation.

Use this dictionary as a faithful friend who will know the answer and never make you feel silly for asking the question! We hope you enjoy your studies and wish you good luck in your endeavours.

The Author Team

Guide to using this book

The term is given in bold.

The pronunciation is in italics

Diamond face shape – *diy-mund fay-s shay-p* – the *head and face shape* determined by a narrow bone structure of the forehead with wide cheekbones tapering to a narrow chin. The ideal hairstyle for this shape is one which minimises the width across the cheekbones. A central *fringe* should be worn with hair full below the cheeks but flat at the cheekbone line. (See head and face shapes on page 161.)

Different needs – *dif-r-unt nee-dz* – differing requirements, especially those of clients. It is illegal to discriminate against clients on grounds of disability, race, ethnicity or sex. See also *client needs, Disability Discrimination Act 1992, 1995 and 2005, Race Relations Act 2000*.

Diffuse alopecia – *dif-yoos alo-pee-sha* – a gradual loss of hair and thinning. Often appearing in women, it is thought to be due to changing *hormone* levels which have a direct affect on *hair follicles*. Pregnancy, the contraceptive pill and the menopause can all contribute to this type of hair loss. It can also be a symptom of some illnesses, such as a thyroid problem or iron

deficiency, so the client should be referred to a *General Practitioner*.

Diffuser – *dif-yooz-ur* – a large plastic attachment, often with prongs, that fits on to a *hairdryer*. It distributes heat so that natural hair movement and curl are encouraged as the hair is dried. The end is placed directly on to the hair where the hair is worked around the fingers in a circular fashion. Being large and open it spreads the heat over a wider section of hair, allowing the hair to be dried slowly and increasing the amount of curl present. See also *finger dry*.

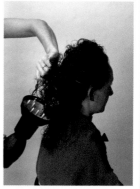

Using a diffuser

Discrepancy d

Diphtheria – *dif-thea-ree-ur* – a highly *contagious* bacterial *infection*. It is a notifiable *disease*, which means it must be reported to the Public Health Authorities by law. It causes a thick grey *membrane* to appear in patches on the skin, which bleeds on removal. The toxins (poisons) from the disease can attack the heart and nerves causing irreparable damage.

Directional perm winding – *diy-rek-shun-ul purm wiyn-ding* – a *directional winding* technique using *perm rods*.

Directional winding – *diy-rek-shun-ul wiyn-ding* – winding *rollers* or *perm rods* into the hair in a specific direction, similar to the way the client will wear the finished hairstyle.

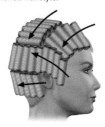

Directional winding

Direct observation – *diy-rekt obs-ur-vay-shun* – the process of directly observing, for example, an *assessor* viewing an *S/NVQ* candidate carrying out tasks which relate to *unit* standards. At times, only parts of a *service* will be observed: for example, when a candidate wishes to be observed for the hair *analysis* and shampooing part of a treatment, but is not yet confident in *cutting* skills. See also *assessment*.

Disability Discrimination Acts 1992, 1995 and 2005 – *dis-u-bil-it-ee dis-krim-in-ay-shun akts* – an Act which states that a person must not discriminate against a person with any disability. In a salon every person has a duty to promote equal opportunities for disabled persons as well as those who are not disabled.

Discount – *dis-k-ow-nt* – money off, or a reduction or mark down in price. See also *calculate*.

Discrepancy – *dis-krep-un-see* – (plural **discrepancies** – *dis-krep-un-seez*) – a difference between items or a disagreement between people's understanding of something.

39

Bold italic words refer to other entries in the book.

Absorption – *ab-saw-p-shun* – the soaking up or taking in of a substance. The skin has the ability to soak up liquids by allowing *molecules* of the right size, such as those in drugs applied to the skin, to penetrate it. Sunlight (in the form of ultra-violet rays) is also absorbed by melanocytes (see *melanin*) within the *epidermis* to make Vitamin D.

Acceptable – *ak-sep-t-ibul* – suitable or able to be agreed on, such as a payment for *services*, or a booking for an *appointment*.

Accessory – *ak-ses-or-ee* – (plural **accessories** – *ak-ses-or-eez*) – an item used to *complement* an overall look. For the hair these can include diamante clips and fascinators, which are very fashionable for weddings instead of wearing hats.

Accident – *ak-si-dent* – an unforeseen event or happening, which may result in injury, damage or even death.

Accidental breakage – *ak-si-den-tul bray-kij* – damage to stock, equipment or working areas which is not intentional, but may cost a salon money to replace or repair. It may also result in harm or injury.

Accreditation of Prior Learning (APL) – *a-kre-di-tay-shun ov priy-er-ler-ning* – credit given for *evidence* of previous learning or work activities which contributes towards a current award. The evidence must be approved by a qualified APL advisor and be valid, i.e. within the last three years. It can include a formal employer's letter stating *ranges* covered or a certificate of achievement in the portfolio. See also *assessment*.

Accredited assessment centre – *a-kre-di-ted a-ses-mnt sen-ta* – a college or centre of learning, approved by an *Awarding Body*, offering *qualifications* to students. Regular visits by *External Verifiers* or inspectors assure the Awarding Body that the centre is *maintaining good practice* and high standards.

Accurate – *ak-yoor-ut* – to be correct or exact, for example, when talking about client details, booking appointments or taking payments.

Acid mantle – *a-sid man-tul* – the mixture of *sebum* and sweat

1

(see *sweat glands*) on the skin's surface, which forms a waterproof barrier and helps to protect the skin against *infection* and *bacteria*. It has a *pH* between 4.5 and 5.5, so it is slightly *acidic*. (See the structure of the skin diagram on page 159.)

Acidic – *a-sid-ik* – having a *pH* lower than 7. See also *pH scale*.

Acknowledge – *ak-no-lij* – to reply or respond to a client's request or payment.

Acne – *ak-nee* – a *condition* of the skin, sometimes with *inflammation*. There are two types – *acne vulgaris* and *acne rosacea* – both of which are easily recognised.

Acne rosacea – *ak-nee row-zay-sha* – a pronounced reddening (*erythema*) of the brow, cheeks and nose resulting from the *capillary* vessels in the skin becoming wider or larger.

Acne vulgaris – *ak-nee vul-gar-is* – a *condition* of the skin, with congested pores causing blackheads, large spots and, if a *bacterial infection* is present, *boils*. This may lead to scarring and pitting

of the skin's surface. It commonly develops in the teenage years and is thought to be influenced by unstable *hormone* levels.

Activator – *ak-ti-vayt-or* – a *styling* liquid, cream or spray used on wet hair to boost movement or *curls* present in the hair. It has a light-to-firm hold and will protect the hair from *atmospheric moisture*.

Active participation – *ak-tiv par-tis-i-pay-shun* – actively doing something. An example is to learn new tasks or skills which will enhance training and professional development.

Adapt – *a-dap-t* – to change or modify, for example, adjusting the *cutting* position for a haircut on a disabled client in a wheelchair.

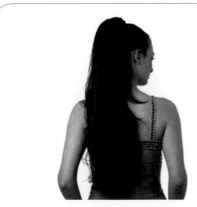

Added hair

Added hair – *a-did hayr* – additional hair that is attached to a client's real hair in the form of hair extensions, wigs or toupees, or clip-on hair pieces.

Add-on service – *ad-on sur-vis* – a **service** which links to another service and can be used to bring in extra money for the salon, whilst giving good value to the client. It provides an opportunity to achieve **productivity targets** for sales.

Adverse – *ad-vurs* – unfavourable, poor or difficult. A **service** may need to be **adapted** for **hair disorders**, **infestations** or **infections** of the hair or skin, **contagious** skin or scalp diseases, and non-infectious conditions. (See infectious diseases of the skin and scalp on pages 162–163.)

Adverse reaction – *ad-vurs ree-ak-shun* – when a client has an unfavourable reaction to a hair or skin test carried out prior to a **perming** or **colouring** service. Sometimes the service cannot be carried out, such as when **metallic salts** are present on the hair, or the client has an **allergic reaction** to the colouring product.

Advertise – *ad-vur-tyz* – to promote, make public or endorse a product or service. For a salon this can include posters, word of mouth, leaflet drops, media publicity on television and radio, and advertising in newspapers and on Internet websites.

Advertising campaign – *ad-vur-tyz-ing cam-payn* – a course of action to increase the number of clients, introduce new **products** and **services**, boost retail sales or promote a forthcoming event for a salon.

Advice – *ad-vyse* – suggestions or **guidance**. For example, recommending **treatments**, **services** or **products** for a client, informing the client on how long a service may take, and giving advance warning to a client, such as preparing the hair by conditioning before a chemical service such as perming or colouring. If a client's request is unrealistic or not suitable for a particular service, this should be stated in a professional manner and an alternative should be given, such as referring the client on to another salon where the service is offered, e.g. when a request is made for **plaiting** Afro-Caribbean hair.

3

Agreement – *a-gree-mnt* – a deal or contract made to gain the client's agreement of the **products** or **services** requested and their costs, before **treatment** starts. The agreement must always meet the client's needs.

Airflow – *ayr-flo* – the direction in which air moves. When using a hairdryer ensure the flow of air is directed from the roots to the tips of the **hair** – that is, in the same direction as the way the **cuticle** scales sit, not against them. This will avoid the cuticle becoming roughened and the hair appearing fluffy and dull.

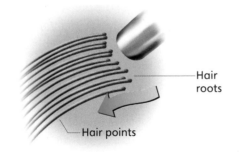

Hair roots

Hair points

Alkaline – *al-ka-lyne* – a substance with a **pH** greater than 7. See also **pH scale.**

Allergic reaction – *a-ler-jik ree-ak-shun* – when a client experiences redness, soreness, swelling or itchiness from the application of a product. The client will not be able to have a full head

colouring service carried out, but may be able to have a service using a **highlighting cap**, as this will provide **protection** and prevent the colouring product making contact with the scalp (known as 'off-scalp application').

Allergy – *a-ler-jee* – (plural **allergies** – *a-ler-jeez*) – an unfavourable reaction to a product. See also **allergic reaction**.

Alopecia – *al-o-pee-sha* – complete or partial **baldness**, which may be congenital (present from birth) or premature (occurring at an early age). Other factors which can bring continued...

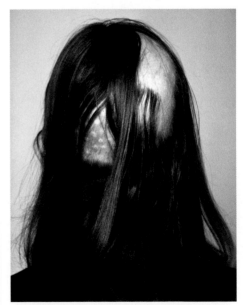

Alopecia

on this condition are the ageing process, emotional stress, certain drugs and **hormone** changes. See also **alopecia areata**.

Alopecia areata – *al-o-pee-sha ar-ee-ay-ta* – bald patches on the crown of the head. The skin is often shiny with frayed hair surrounding the patch. The causes are not fully understood, but it is thought to be an inherited condition and can be brought on by stress or shock. If it distresses the client then referral to a **trichologist** would be advised.

Alopecia totalis – *al-o-pee-sha to-tar-lis* – **baldness** affecting all **terminal hair**, especially the eyebrows, eyelashes, scalp and body hair. Shock has been known to cause total baldness.

Alpha keratin – *al-fa ker-a-tin* – dry, un-stretched hair in its natural **state**, before it is **set** or **blow-dried**. See also **beta keratin**.

Alternative – *awl-tur-na-tiv* – another option or choice, for example, to **refer** a client to another salon which specialises in the client's needs.

Anagen – *an-a-jen* – the most active period of the **hair growth cycle** when the cells of the **dermal papilla** reproduce actively to form new hairs. At any one time 90% of the hair on the head will be in this stage. If a person's hair has a long anagen phase, the hair can grow to a long length; for people whose hair has a short anagen phase their hair cannot grow long. (See the hair growth cycle diagram on page 160.)

Analyse – *an-a-l-yze* – to study or examine something in detail in order to discover more about it.

Analysis – *a-nal-i-sis* – a full assessment of the **condition** of the hair and scalp, by doing a **visual check** and by manual testing, to ensure there are no factors which would prevent a **service** from taking place. It is also done to give the best treatment **advice** to the client. Any problems found should be dealt with promptly and in the correct, **professional** manner, informing a **line manager**, and if an **infectious** disease has been identified, telling other **colleagues**. See also **necessary tests**, **contraindication**, **contra-action**, **medical referral**.

Androgenic alopecia – *an-dro-je-nic al-o-pee-sha* – *male pattern baldness* with a receding hairline at the front and a thinning of the crown. Eventually the whole head is left with short, soft, downy hair. This condition is passed on through families on the male side. Many men prefer to have a *clipper cut* using a *grade* 1 or 2 to even out the effect.

Angle – *an-gul* – the direction in which hair is held in order for it to be cut or wound on to a *roller* or *perm rod*. For example, hair which is held directly out from the head is said to be at a 90 degree angle.

Antibiotic – *an-tee-by-yo-tik* – a medicine which destroys *bacteria*, used to clear an *infection*. For a skin disease, this treatment is given either orally, injected into the muscle or applied straight on to the skin.

Anticipate others' needs – *an-ti-si-pay-t u-thurz nee-dz* – to foresee what other people might need. For example, if a senior *stylist* asks a junior member of staff to assist with a colour service, the assistant will know that a protective apron and gloves are needed and the client will need a colouring gown and towel.

Anti-oxidant – *an-tee-ox-i-dnt* – properties within some conditioners used after chemical processes to reduce the amount of chemical residue left in the hair.

Appearance – *ap-eer-untz* – how something or someone looks. A salon *employee* should appear *professional*, not only for *health and safety* reasons but to give the correct impression to the client. For an *S/NVQ* candidate, it is part of the *assessment* criteria, so if the candidate's appearance is less than professional, he or she may be graded as non-competent after the assessment.

Application by brush – *ap-li-kay-shun biy br-ush* – applying a product by using a lather brush. For a *shaving service*, a bristle brush is used to lather up shaving products and apply them to the face.

Application by massage – *ap-li-kay-shun biy mas-arj* – applying a product using the hands. This is essential to do in a *shaving service*, if the area to be worked on is too small to use a lather brush.

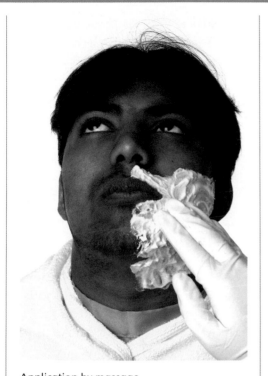
Application by massage

Appointment details – *a-poynt-mnt dee-tay-ls* – all relevant information about an **appointment** that needs to be recorded: client's name and contact details, the service required, the date and time of the appointment, staff booked to perform the **service** and estimated length of time required. See also **appointments system**.

Appointments system – *a-poynt-mnts sis-tum* – a method for booking **appointments**, whereby the **booking details** are either written into an appointment book or typed into a computerised electronic programme, usually tailored for the salon. Staff need to be trained in the salon's particular system for it to work successfully. See also **Data Protection Act 1998**.

Applicator bottle – *ap-li-kay-tur bot-ul* – a bottle used for mixing **quasi-permanent colour** products as they are more runny in nature than **permanent colour**, **high lift tints** or **bleach**. It is used for quick application techniques.

Appointment – *a-poynt-mnt* – a date and time placed in a booking-in sheet stating the name of the client, the type of **service** requested and the **stylist** who will be providing the service. See also **appointment details**.

Appraisal – *a-pray-zul* – a judgement or review of the effectiveness of equipment or staff. It is usually carried out by a **line manager**, at a mutually agreed time, with set aims and objectives, which results in a professional development plan being set up for future training and development.

Approachable – *a-pro-chu-bul* – friendly and easy to continued...

7

talk to. It is important that clients feel they are able to approach an *employee* in a salon and can expect good customer service. A *stylist* who is unapproachable will lose clients very quickly!

Appropriate – *a-pro-pree-ut* – suitable or fit for the situation, such as using correct spoken language, suitable body language, a *professional* manner when dealing with clients, and choosing the best time to sell products or *services*.

Apron – *ay-prun* – a protective garment worn during chemical processes to avoid staining clothes.

Arrector pili muscles – *a-rek-tor pi-li mus-suls* – minute, smooth muscles of the skin, attached to the *hair follicles*. Classed as involuntary muscles, they are not under the control of a person's conscious thought. For example, when the temperature becomes very cold, the muscles contract causing the hair follicles to stand up straight. The skin has the effect of 'goose bumps'. This helps to keep in heat under the skin. (See the structure of the skin diagram on page 159.)

Assertive – *as-ur-tiv* – being confident and self-assured, but not arrogant or forceful. It enables you to be protective of your own rights in your job role whilst supporting others.

Assess – *a-ses* – to *evaluate* or determine the quality of something.

Assessment – *a-ses-mnt* – *evidence* using a variety of methods to show that a candidate is competent in an area of study. Usually there are several methods depending on the qualification sought. All assessment books show the following evidence codes, regardless of the *Awarding Body*:

x1 observed work

x2 witness statements

x3 assessments of prior learning and experience (APL)

x4 oral questions

x5 written questions and/or assignments

x6 other forms of evidence (e.g. photographic).

Assessor – *a-ses-ur* – a person with an assessing *qualification* who is employed by a centre or *Awarding Body* to help a candidate understand the *evidence* required of them and work through the *assessment* process. Assessors ensure that the evidence provided by the candidate covers all areas of competence required. They should be fair and able to make sound and consistent judgements about the acceptability of evidence.

Assistance – *a-sis-tens* – help, aid or support to colleagues, clients or people making enquiries. Being *courteous*, polite and *professional* is essential and it will help you to learn new skills, e.g., offering to assist senior *stylists* with advanced treatments.

Atmospheric moisture – *at-mus-fe-ric moy-s-cha* – moisture that is found within the air, such as steam from hot baths, fog, rain or damp air. It changes hair from a *beta keratin* state back to *alpha keratin* (natural state).

Atom – *a-tum* – the smallest unit of matter, of which everything is made up.

Attachment technique – *a-ta-ch-mnt tek-nee-k* – a method of applying *hair extensions* to a client's real hair. See also *added hair*.

Authorisation – *or-thu-riy-zay-shun* – consent or approval to do something. Official permission from a supervisor or a person in management is often needed to perform a treatment, carry out payments or sell gift vouchers. Also, when making a payment, a client needs to authorise use of his or her credit or debit card by entering the authorisation code or PIN number in the machine.

Avant-garde – *a-vont-gard* – an image which is the forerunner of fashion, or the development of a hairstyle beyond what is commercially acceptable (acceptable styles worn by the average person and commonly known as high street fashion). This style is usually too extravagant to be worn as an everyday hairstyle.

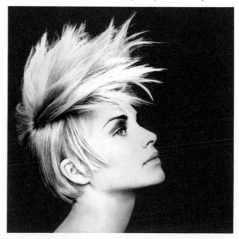

An avant-garde style

9

Award – *a-wor-d* – a collection of completed (and assessed) units which covers sufficient *evidence* to allow accreditation for a *qualification*.

Awarding Body (AB) – *a-wor-ding bo-dee* – a top-level training organisation whose name and logo appear on certificates. It does not deliver the training, but designs and accredits the *qualification* used by colleges and assessment centres. An Awarding Body must be inspected and approved by the Qualifications and Curriculum Authority (QCA) – a government body which ensures qualifications are fair and obtainable. All Awarding Bodies comply with the *National Occupational Standards (NOS)*, so the qualification for each Awarding Body is equal whichever one is taken. There are several Awarding Bodies within the Hairdressing and Beauty Therapy industry, such as:

- Vocational Training Charitable Trust (VTCT)
- City and Guilds (C & G)
- International Training and Examining Council (ITEC)
- Edexcel
- Scottish Qualifications Authority (SQA).

Backbrushing – *bak br-ush-ing* – see *backcombing*

Backcombing – *bak ko-ming* – matting the hair together in a controlled manner to give body, lift, support and hold to a hair style. The technique involves taking a *mesh of hair* and pushing the hair back towards the root. The amount of times this is done determines the amount of backcombing that is put into the hair. This creates a supporting pad of hair at the roots. Doing this on the whole *length* of hair creates *volume* which helps to pad out finer hair. It is often used to add volume to hair-up styles.

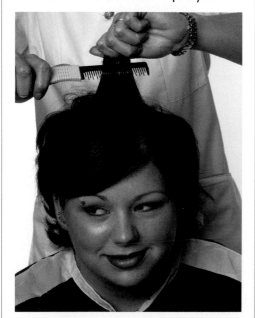

Backcombing

Backwash basin – *bak wosh bays-in* – a wash basin commonly used in salons for shampooing hair to prevent water and chemicals entering the client's eyes and the clothes from getting wet. The client should be positioned right back in the seat so that the neck fits in the curve of the basin correctly, without any gaps for water to leak through.

Bacteria – *bak-ter-ee-a* – one-celled *micro-organisms*, visible only under a microscope. They are classified by their shape, and need food, oxygen, warmth and darkness to grow and multiply. The presence of bacterial *infections* is a *contraindication* to a *service* and a *medical referral* should be advised. Most infections respond well to *antibiotics*.

Bactericide – *bak-ter-i-syde* – any agent that destroys *bacteria*, such as bacitracin – an antibiotic used to treat *infections* of the skin, outer ear and eyelids. The saliva produced in the mouth, and tears from the eyes, also have antibacterial properties to prevent infection. Disinfectant in liquid form (usually *Barbicide*®) is used to kill the majority of bacteria, *infestations* and *fungi* in salons, but *sterilisation* is needed continued...

to destroy **viruses**, spores and more resistant strains of bacteria. Simple hand washing with a disinfectant soap will prevent the build-up of bacteria on the hands and the spread of germs.

Baggy ends – b-ag-ee enz – when hair falls off the side of a **roller** or **perm rod**, because the size of the section being taken is too large for the size of the roller or rod. This creates an uneven **curl** formation.

Balance – bal-uns – in equal **proportion**, for example, whether the **lengths** of hair are even throughout. It is important to assess the balance for the finished result of a set, blow-dry or a hair-up style.

Baldness – borl-d-nes – the absence of hair on all or part of the scalp. See also **alopecia**.

Banding – ban-ding – a band of colour different from the rest of the hair. This occurs if fresh colour is applied over existing artificial colour (overlapping) during a **re-growth application** of colour.

Bantu knot – ban-too not – see **twist**.

Barbering – bar-bur-ing – the name given to men's hairdressing services.

Barber's rash – bar-burs ra-sh – **inflammation** of the **hair follicles** in the beard area, caused by bacterial **infection**, resulting in **pustules** forming and scabbing of the skin. Also called **barber's itch**. See also **folliculitis**, **infection**.

Barbicide® – bar-bi-syde – a type of disinfectant in liquid form, often used in salons to kill **bacteria**, **infestations** and **fungi**.

Barrel curl – ba-rel kur-l – a soft-centred **curl**. It creates loose, springy curls that stand away from the head. See also **pin curling**.

Barrier cream – bar-ee-a kreem – a cream applied around the hairline during **perming** and **colouring** to prevent irritation or burning, and staining of the skin. It is available in various forms. Petroleum jelly can also be used.

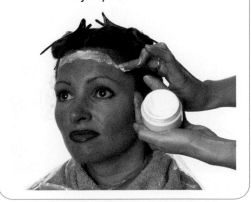

Basal layer – *bay-sul lay-ur* – the last and deepest layer of the *epidermis* of the skin, which lies on top of the *dermis*. It consists of living 'parent' cells which reproduce constantly to make new cells called keratinocytes. Keratinocytes produce the protein *keratin*, which strengthens all the cells of hair, skin and nails. (See the structure of the skin diagram on page 159.)

Base colour – *bay-s kul-ur* – see *depth*.

Basic skills – *bay-sik sk-ilz* – the skills needed to read, write and use maths at a basic level so that a person can function and progress, both at work and in society. They are often used to gain a key skill certificate in numeracy, literacy or computer skills, which helps to achieve other qualifications such as *S/NVQs*.

Beard clippings – *b-eerd k-lip-ings* – pieces of hair that have been cut away from a beard. A client needs to be correctly gowned so that these cuttings do not come in contact with the client's skin and clothes and cause discomfort.

Beard trim – *b-eerd t-rim* – to cut facial hair growing on the chin, cheek and neck area. The natural growth and *density* of the hair determine the shape of the beard and which *cutting* techniques to use.

Behaviour – *bu-hayv-yoor* – actions or deeds, conduct, manner or performance. Salon behaviour should be *positive* and *professional*, especially when delivering *services* and *selling* products, but also because it generates a good atmosphere within the salon.

Benefit – *ben-if-it* – an advantage. For example, using a conditioner helps the *cuticle* to lie flat, thereby giving the hair a shiny appearance.

Benefits of products – *ben-if-its ov pro-duk-ts* – *selling* points that reflect the best features of products. They are the advantages to a client when using that product.

Beta keratin – *bee-ta ker-a-tin* – hair that has been stretched and allowed to cool into a new shape. This occurs after *setting* or *blow-drying*.

Bleach – *b-lee-ch* – a *gel*, cream or powder which lightens the hair and has the ability to lift out most *colouring* products. When it is applied to dry hair it changes *melanin* into a colourless oxy-melanin (see *oxidation*). Seven levels of lift can be achieved which means this product will not wash out of the hair.

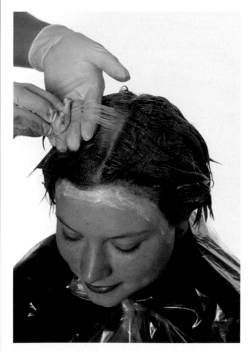

Removing bleach to check the colour match from roots to ends

Bleaching – *b-lee-ch-ing* – the process of applying *bleach*.

Blend in – *b-lend in* – to join sections of natural and synthetic (man-made) hair together when adding hair so they are no longer separate. The aim is to achieve a good colour and size match between the two types of hair. See also *yarn locks* and *silky locks*.

Block colour – *blok kul-ur* – a colour applied to sections of hair. It is applied using the same method as a *full head application*.

Blood – *blu-d* – the red fluid circulating through the body, pumped by the heart, carried away from the heart in arteries, and brought back to the heart via the veins. It contains blood cells which provide nourishment and oxygen to the cells of the body and takes away all waste products. Arteries bring oxygen and nutrients to the cells of the *dermis* via the *capillaries*. Waste products are collected from the skin and returned via the capillaries to the veins. The blood supply can be increased to any area through massage or other stimulation of the arteries, veins and capillaries. For example, a scalp massage will increase the blood flow to the *hair shaft* and the skin, encouraging growth and repair of the tissue.

Blood supply (to the hair) – *blu-d sup-liy* – the supply of **blood** to the hair, entering the papilla in the **dermis**. It brings nutrients to nourish and feed the cells, provides oxygen, then takes away the waste products. This keeps the hair healthy and encourages growth and repair to cells which may be damaged. (See the structure of the skin diagram on page 159.)

Blow-dry – *b-low driy* – to remove moisture from the hair, using a hand-held electrical **hairdryer**. Various **styling** tools and **equipment** are used to re-form the hair into its new shape. The hair's structure allows this process to take place by the breaking down and re-forming of **hydrogen bonds**. See also **airflow** and **straightening**.

Body language – *bo-dee lang-wij* – unconscious or automatic body or hand gestures, facial expressions or body movements which reflect how a person is feeling. It can reveal confidence, or lack of it, and moods and emotions. See also **personal space**.

Body heat – *bod-ee heet* – heat given off by the body.

Boil – *boy-ul* – an acute **inflammation** surrounding a **hair follicle** caused by bacterial **infection**. It can be very painful and may require drainage or lancing and a course of **antibiotics**. See also **infection**.

Bond – *bon-d* – to bind or hold things together, for example, applying **hair extensions** using a type of glue to secure them to existing hair.

Booking details – *bu-king dee-t-aylz* – necessary information given by a client in order to make an appointment for a **service**. See also **appointment details**.

Braid – *b-rayd* – a form of **plait**, where the hair is woven and secured by using suitable bands. It can be a **scalp plait**, **corn row** or a combination of plaits.

Brick perm winding – *br-ik pur-m wiyn-ding* – winding **perm rods** into the hair to create a brick wall effect. The first rod is placed at the front hairline and the section behind this roller is divided in the middle where the next two rollers are placed. This pattern is used both in **setting** and *continued…*

15

perming, as it directs the hair away from the face without creating any *partings* in the hair. It is a useful technique for fine hair.

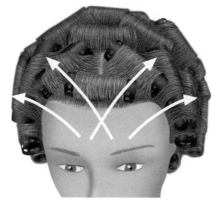

Brick perm winding

Budget – *bud-jit* – an allotted sum of money available for spending. It is usually set out as a *plan* showing the proposed outgoings of the salon. Keeping regular reports will help to avoid overspending. See also *overheads*.

Budgetary constraint – *bud-jit-ury kon-strayn-tz* – a *restriction* on the amount of money for spending. For example, when organising a *hair show* or event a *budget* will need to be drawn up and adhered to.

Build-up – *bil-d-up* – an accumulation of something, for example, when some hair *products*, such as hairspray, cling to the *hair shaft* over time, making the hair appear dull and lifeless. This creates a barrier to performing other hairdressing *services* on the hair. See also *clarifying shampoo*.

Business plan – *biz-nes pl-an* – a written outline covering all aspects of the business, including start-up costs, the type and location of the business, the resources required to run it, *cash flow prediction*, staffing expectations and the growth and development of the business over a set period – usually five years. A bank or financial backer would need to see one before agreeing to invest money into the business. Most banks provide support and a blank business plan to fill in, prior to a meeting with the bank manager.

Buying signals – *b-iy-ing s-ig-n-uls* – signs indicating that a client is interested in buying a *product* or wanting a *service* to be carried out. They can include engaging in a conversation and asking questions about the product or service, enquiring about prices, actively listening and making eye contact. It is important for a salon employee to recognise these to avoid missing out on a *sale*. See also *selling*.

Calculate – *kal-kyoo-layt* – to work out the amount of something, for example, a payment due. An example is when a salon offers special promotions or discounts given to regular clients, such as 10% off a service.

Candidate – *can-did-ayt* – a person working towards achieving a **qualification**. A life-time registration number is issued by an **Awarding Body** which is always used, regardless of how many qualifications are being sought.

Capillary – *kap-i-lur-ee* – (plural **capillaries** – *kap-i-lur-eez*) – a small **blood** vessel designed to supply nutrients to cells.

Cash – *k-ash* – money given in exchange for **services** and **products**. It should be **legal tender**, i.e. notes or coins of the country in which the salon is based.

Cash equivalent – *k-ash u-kwiv-u-lunt* – equal in value to cash. This is usually in the form of a gift voucher, pre-paid by the person giving the voucher and used by the person who has received the gift voucher. The till and payment system used is exactly the same as for cash, and the voucher is counted in the takings at the end of the day during the **cashing up** session.

Cash flow prediction – *k-ash flo pru-dik-shun* – a guide or estimate of all the monies that will be required over a set period to meet the demands of a business. It helps to see the balance between revenue coming in and money paid out.

Cash point – *k-ash p-oynt* – a dispensing point for money. Customers insert their debit or credit card into the machine, along with their personal identification number (PIN) for security, to withdraw money, providing there are available funds.

Cashing up – *k-ash-ing up* – counting the till money at the end of the business day. The amount should marry up with the **takings** sheet, recording sales and the treatment page for bookings. Once the **float** has been put back into the till for the next day, the takings are recorded and placed into a safe, or taken to the bank.

Catagen – *kat-a-jin* – part of the *hair growth cycle*, when the *dermal papilla* separates from the *matrix* and the *hair follicle* begins to break down. Gradually, the hair becomes detached from the follicle. Often referred to as the transitional phase, meaning going from one phase to another. (See the hair growth cycle diagram on page 160.)

Chemotherapy – *kee-mo-ther-a-pee* – a medical treatment for *disease*, especially of cancer, using chemical substances. It is a *contraindication* to some scalp massage techniques, such as *high frequency* treatments.

Cheque – *ch-e-k* – a form of payment provided by banks,

Channel setting – *chan-ul set-ing* – a uniform *setting* technique whereby *rollers* are placed in a line beginning from the front hairline working to the *nape* and then in two channels both sides of the middle section. This pattern is used in *wet setting*. This is the first setting technique that is taught to students as it helps to work out how the rollers fit into the shape of the head. When **dressed out** it produces a uniform look with the hair directed back from the forehead and down at the sides and back.

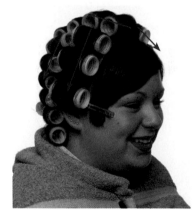

Channel setting technique

Chemical service – *kem-i-kul sur-vis* – a *process* carried out on a client that involves the use of chemicals which affects the structure of the hair such as *perming*, *straightening* and *colouring*. See also *under-processing*, *over-processing*.

largely overtaken by the use of credit and debit cards. The payee (name of the person or company who is receiving the payment) and the amount of money being paid is written on the cheque, dated then signed. A bank card should be shown alongside the continued...

cheque to provide extra security. The card details are then recorded on the back.

Cicatricial alopecia – *sik-a-tri-shul al-o-pee-sha* – loss of hair over *scar tissue* within the skin, caused by burns, wounds or *infection* in the area. Very little can be done, but if the client wishes to be referred on, a *trichologist* can advise. If the *hair follicle* has been destroyed there is little hope of hair regrowing. A transplant or plugs of hair may be inserted into the skin.

Circular brush – *sur-kyoo-lur br-ush* – a brush used for producing a curled effect in the hair. Wet hair is moulded around the cylinder of the brush and dried with a *hairdryer* to create a curled look. The smaller the brush, the tighter the *curl* will be.

Circulation problems – *sur-kyoo-lay-shun prob-lumz* – see *heart problems*.

Clarifying shampoo – *klar-if-iy-ing sham-poo* – a type of *shampoo* used for removing *build-up* of *products* on the hair, such as *hair spray*. It strips the hair of these products helping to reduce product residue.

Classic look – *kla-sik luk* – a hairstyle that never dates or goes out of fashion. It is a look which is timeless, for example, the one-length bob haircut.

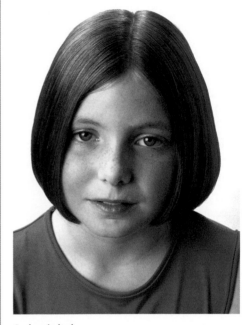

A classic bob

Clear layer – *klee-r lay-ur* – the second layer within the *epidermis* of the skin, below the *horny layer*. This layer is composed of dead, flattened cells which are found on the soles of the feet and palms of the hand to protect them from wear and tear. (See the structure of the skin diagram on page 159.)

Client – *kl-iy-unt* – a person who pays for *services* or *products* offered within a salon.

Client care – *kl-iy-unt k-ayr* – looking after the client, in the most *professional* manner possible, so that the client gains maximum benefit from the *service* and wishes to return to the salon.

Client commitment – *kl-iy-unt kom-it-mnt* – an agreement by a client to book a *service*, such as a particular treatment, or course of specialist or corrective treatments, or to purchase a *product*.

Client expectations – *kl-iy-unt ex-pekt-ay-shunz* – beliefs by the client that he or she will receive a high standard of care and the necessary *professional* services to satisfy the client's needs. If the expectations are unrealistic, then advice and guidance must be given. For example, if the client wants a celebrity-type hairstyle, but it would be unsuitable for the client's *head and face shape* and hair texture, then it is up to the stylist to dissuade the client, giving reasons tactfully. See also *client needs*.

Client experience – *kl-iy-unt ex-peer-ee–uns* – the observations made by the client. The client should be delighted with the finished results of a *service*.

Client groups – *kl-iy-unt groops* – types of clients and their ethnic hair properties. The Commission for Racial Equality (CRE) breaks these groups down into White, Mixed, Black, Asian and Chinese.

Client needs – *kl-iy-unt needz* – the wishes of the client, based on *client expectations*. It is important that these are met to the best of the hairdresser's *professional* ability. However, after a full *consultation*, if the requested *service* or treatment is not suitable for the client, then the client should be told in an honest way and an alternative suggested.

Client record – *kl-iy-unt rek-ord* – full details of a client's personal and *contact details*, including *services* carried out on the client. Written on cards or inputted on the computer, this *confidential* information should include dates of services, any adverse reactions to hair *continued...*

testing carried out and personal preferences for **products**. Adding details which help with customer relations and prevent embarrassment is encouraged. For example, if a client has recently been widowed this information will help a new stylist to avoid asking after the client's spouse. See also **Data Protection Act 1998**.

Client requirements – kl-iy-unt ru-kwiy-r-mnts – the **services** or treatments to be given to a client after **client needs** and expectations have been discussed during a **consultation** with the stylist.

Client rights – kl-iy-unt riy-ts – the legal rights of a client which are protected by law. See also **Consumer Protection Act 1987**, **Consumer Safety Act 1978**, **Cosmetic Products (Safety) Regulations 2004**.

Client satisfaction – kl-iy-unt sat-is-fak-shun – fulfilment of **client expectations** to the best of a hairdresser's **professional** ability.

Client's features – kl-iy-unts fee-churz – distinguishing aspects, such as the **head and** **face shape**, and shape and size of the client's eyes, nose and ears, which need to be taken into account when **cutting** and **styling** the client's hair.

Client's lifestyle – kl-iy-unts liy-f-stiy-l – a client's way of life, habits, daily grooming routine, such as how he or she maintains the hairstyle at home. Careful questioning during the **consultation** will provide these answers.

Climazone – kl-iy-ma-zown – electrical **equipment** that provides added heat to speed up colour developing time. Found in various shapes and sizes, its 'arms' can be turned off if not required, so that specific areas of the head can be targeted.

Clipper attachments – klip-ur ut-ach-mnts – sometimes called **grades**, these are fittings which are attached to the cutting head of **clippers** in order to cut the hair to a specific **length**. The higher the number is on the grade, the longer the hair will be left. For example, a Grade 1 attachment is the shortest and will cut very close to the scalp, Grades 2–4 *continued...*

will leave the hair short, whereas Grades 5–8 will leave the hair longer. They should not be used if they have missing or broken teeth as this will result in an uneven haircut.

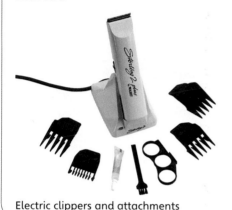

Electric clippers and attachments

Clipper cut – *klip-ur kut* – a cut done with *clippers*, especially on men's hair.

Clipper-over-comb – *klip-ur-o-vur-ko-m* – a *cutting* method used with *clippers* and a *cutting comb*. Hair is combed out from the head and held within the comb while the clippers are used to cut off the hair protruding from the comb. The technique is ideal for hair that is too short to hold, for *tapering* hair into the hairline or neck, or getting in difficult-to-reach areas.

Clippers – *klip-ur-z* – electrical *equipment* used for *beard trims* and to cut dry hair to a very short *length*. *Clipper attachments* are fitted which determine the length of the finished cut. Available as a re-chargeable unit, the clippers sit on a base and can be used without wires or cords that may otherwise get in the way.

Clockspring curl – *klok-sp-ring kur-l* – a *curl* which sits flat on the head with a closed middle. It is looser at the roots, gradually getting tighter towards the ends. See also *pin curling*.

Closed questions – *klo-zd kwes-chun-z* – *questions* requiring a 'yes' or 'no' answer only. *continued...*

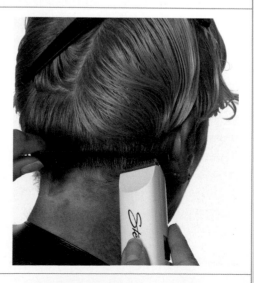

Sometimes they need to be asked during a **consultation**, but, generally, closed questions stop a conversation from flowing and should be avoided. See also **open questions**.

Closing a sale – k-lo-zing u s-ayl – gaining a firm commitment by the client to buy a **product** or book a **service**. See also **buying signals**, **selling**.

Club cutting – kl-ub kut-ing – a **cutting** technique which leaves the ends of the hair blunt, removing **length** only. This method is used universally and will help to give the hair a thicker appearance as the ends are blunt.

Code of Practice – k-owd ov prak-tis – this is not a piece of legislation, that is, it not a legal requirement. However, all professional organisations have a Code of Practice, as do most salons. It is a guideline to correct procedures and etiquette (**behaviour**) to follow for all aspects of treatment, which promotes safe practice. It underpins the legal Acts supporting the health and safety of everyone within the workplace. When a therapist or stylist joins a professional membership, they

sign to say they abide by the organisation's Code of Practice. Failure to uphold good practice may affect the **insurance** cover offered by the organisation and may result in **negligence**, leaving the stylist open to prosecution.

Collating – ko-layt-ing – gathering together information. It is useful to store information in a logical and safe location. For **S/NVQ** candidates, using spreadsheets and database programs on a computer will allow them to present findings in an interesting way. Other information in a variety of formats (worksheets, practical demonstrations, images) can also be combined for a presentation or an **assessment**.

Colleague – kol-ee-g – a co-worker employed in a salon – from the receptionist to a member of senior staff. Also refers to a fellow member of a profession.

Colour correction – kul-ur kor-ek-shun – making good problems that have occurred as a result of a **colouring** service. Examples include removing artificial colour that is too dark and removing **banding** of colours that continued...

has been caused by the overlapping of the *product* during a *re-growth application*.

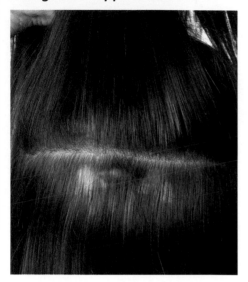

A case for colour correction

Colour mapping – *kul-ur mapping* – placing colours in the hair to emphasise a haircut, make the hair appear longer or shorter or denser, or to add texture. For example, placing a lighter colour in the *nape* of shoulder length hair gives the *appearance* of longer looking hair, while darker colours give the impression of adding *density* to the hair.

Colour remover – *kul-ur rumoo-vur* – a product that strips or removes artificial colour from the hair. It is not always possible to remove all colour completely, if the hair has been coloured over a length of time and has a very dark *base colour*.

Colour spectrum – *kul-ur spektrum* – the range of colours that make up white sunlight, as seen in a rainbow: red, orange, yellow, green, blue, indigo, violet.

Colour wheel – *kul-ur wee-l* – a circle divided into six equal portions made up from the three *primary colours* – red, yellow and blue. The primary colours, when mixed, form the secondary colours – orange, green and violet. These colours are then split into warm tones (red, orange and yellow) and cool tones (green, blue and violet). The wheel is used to help find *neutralising* tones or to replace missing tones in the hair, by identifying the opposite colour on the colour continued...

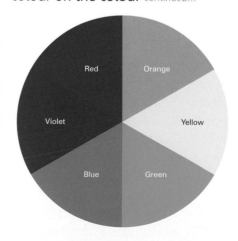

wheel. For example, if the hair has too much red (warmth) in it, a colour that contained green (ash tone) would be used to neutralise some of the unwanted warmth in the colour.

Colouring – *kul-ur-ing* – the process of adding *temporary colour*, *quasi-permanent colour* or *permanent colour* to a client's hair. See also *bleaching* and *high lift tint*.

Comb twist – *ko-m tw-ist* – see *twisting*.

Commercially viable – *kom-ur-shal-ee viy-ubul* – realistic and achievable in a business sense; making a *profit*. Booking a client in for a perm, cut and style within an hour and charging five pounds for the service is not *cost effective*. See also *commercially viable time*.

Commercially viable time – *kom-ur-shal-ee viy-ubul tiym* – the specific, realistic and *cost effective* time allocated to performing a service within a salon. For *S/NVQ assessment* purposes, times have been laid down by the Qualifications and Curriculum Authority (QCA). These times must be adhered to and assessors are not allowed to pass assessments if a service takes longer than the specific time allowed.

Commission – *kom-i-shun* – a reward or incentive given to stylists selling products, performing services or increasing business in some way. See also *targets*.

Compatible – *kom-pat-u-bul* – suitable, such as *products* or *services* that can be used together without problems.

Competence – *kom-put-tuns* – the ability to perform a set task, to a particular standard. For an *S/NVQ* candidate it shows knowledge and understanding of the subject, full awareness of the task and related *health and safety* issues. *Evidence* of competence in a *range* or *performance criteria* can be gained in several units simultaneously. For example, in one service the candidate may carry out: hair analysis and shampooing (Unit G7/G9), actual service (Unit H6), selling of related products (Unit G6).

Competition judges – *kom-put-i-shun ju-jez* – respected members of an industry who examine and assess *competition work* critically.

Competition work – *kom-put-i-shun werk* – work carried out in an in-house, regional, national or international competition. Hairstyles are practised to perfection and then produced at a specific venue under various conditions and restraints (for example, only being allowed a specific amount of time).

Competitive – *kom-pet-u-tiv* – trying to gain business over other businesses in the same field. Knowing how to attract clients away from other hairdressing salons is an example of competing in a competitive market.

Complaint – *kom-play-nt* – a *grievance* or criticism, in particular, as a result of a client being dissatisfied. A complaints procedure as stated by the salon rules should be followed and any complaint should be treated in a *professional* and calm manner. Too many complaints indicate that the business is not functioning as it should and clients are less likely to return. See also *client satisfaction*, *client expectations*, *client needs*, *client rights*.

Complement – *kom-pl-mnt* – to enhance, for example, adding

accessories to a hairstyle to complete a desired look.

Concise – *kon-s-iys* – accurate, to the point.

Conclusion – *kon-cloo-shun* – a final result or summary.

Condition – *kon-di-shun* – the state of something. This refers not only to hair – the state of which can be determined by manual testing as well as examining *test results* – but also to products sold. For example, products sold to clients must not be damaged. See also *Sale of Goods Act 1979*, *Supply of Goods and Services Act 1982*.

Conditioner – *kon-di-shun-ur* – a product applied to the hair to make it smoother, softer and more manageable. See also *surface conditioner*, *penetrating conditioner*, *scalp treatment*.

Conditioning – *kon-di-shun-ing* – improving the condition of the hair, by applying *conditioner*, to make it more manageable and to *enhance* its *appearance*.

Conditioning massage techniques – *kon-di-shun-ing mas-arj tek-neeks* – *continued...*

massage movements used when *conditioning* hair, such as *effleurage* and *petrissage*.

Confidential – *kon-fi-den-shul* – private, not to be shared. See also *client record* and *Data Protection Act 1998*.

Consequence – *kon-si-kw-ens* – an outcome or a result of an action. For example, potential side effects of hair extensions, if problems occur, are hair loss or *traction alopecia*.

Constructive recommendation – *kon-stru-kt-iv rek-om-en-day-shun* – a *positive*, helpful suggestion.

Consultation – *kon-sul-tay-shun* – a discussion between a *stylist* and a client to determine the services and treatments that reflect *client requirements*.

Consumer legislation – *kon-syoo-mur lej-is-lay-shun* – see *client rights*, *Consumer Protection Act 1987*, *Consumer Safety Act 1978*, *Cosmetic Products (Safety) Regulations 2004* and all *legislation* under the *Sale of Goods Act 1979*.

Consumer Protection Act 1987 – *kon-syoo-mur pro-tek-shun akt* – this Act safeguards the consumer against:

- defective products
- injuries sustained from defective products
- misleading prices.

Consumer Safety Act 1978 – *kon-syoo-mur say-f-tee akt* – this Act requires a business to reduce the possible risk to consumers from any product that may be potentially dangerous.

Contact details – *kon-t-akt dee-t-aylz* – personal information, such as postal address, e-mail address and phone numbers. Taking down a client's telephone or mobile phone number allows the client to be notified should a change of booking be required.

Contact dermatitis – see *dermatitis*.

Contagious – *kon-tay-jus* – transmitted (of disease) from one person to another, by direct or indirect contact. See also *infections*, *folliculitis*, *impetigo*, *scabies* and infectious diseases of the skin and scalp on pages 162–163.

Continuing professional development (CPD) – *kon-tin-yoo-ing pru-fe-shun-ul du-vel-up-mnt* – ongoing personal training, to keep up-to-date with techniques and new trends within an industry. This ensures that the skills of *S/NVQ* candidates remain current and increases their chances of becoming employed. *Assessors* and *Internal Verifiers* are expected to have a CPD folder showing courses and additional training with points allotted to them. The candidate's *Awarding Body* should be referred to for the points system used. When going for an interview, it is important for the candidate to have a CPD folder, which includes *qualifications* and *evidence*, to show a prospective employer.

Contra-action – *kon-tra-ak-shun* – a mild or severe reaction to a service or procedure which may require a *medical referral*. An example is an *allergic reaction* to chemicals in hair dye. See also *adverse reaction*.

Contract of employment – *kon-tra-kt ov em-ploy-mnt* – a written agreement between a person and an employer stating full job responsibilities and conditions of service including: working area,

salary payment, holiday entitlement, *health and safety* responsibilities, and which line manager to report to. See also *job role*.

Contractor – *kon-tra-kt-ur* – a person or firm who supplies materials, labour or specialist skills to a business.

Contractual agreement – *kon-tra-kt-yoo-ul u-gree-mnt* – an agreement of legal rights between a person, such as a client, and a salon, drawn up as a written contract. Examples include a deposit on a course of treatments or an order for the purchase of electrical *equipment*. See also *legislation*.

Contraindication – *kon-tra-in-di-kay-shun* – any reason that prevents a service or treatment from taking place, such as the presence of a *disease*, *hair disorder* or *infestation* of the scalp or *infection* of the skin, or breakage to the hair. For example, if head lice are present there is a risk of *cross-infection* within a salon.

Control measure – *kon-trol mes-yoor* – an action which can be taken to reduce or *continued...*

manage a person's *risk* to *health and safety*. (See legislation on pages 164–165.)

Control of Substances Hazardous to Health Regulations 2002 (COSHH) – *kon-tro-l ov sub-stn-siz ha-zur-dus too hel-th reg-yoo-lay-shunz* – These regulations require employers to:

- control people's exposure to hazardous substances in the workplace
- identify, list and assess in writing any substance in the workplace
- ensure control measures are in place for hazardous and other substances in the workplace.

Controlling risks – *kon-tro-l-ing ri-s-ks* – checking and limiting the possibility of harm occurring by identifying and minimising *risks*, and ensuring safe practice within the salon. (See legislation on pages 164–165.)

Cool tones – *kool to-nz* – colours that contain violet, blue or green.

Cool towel – *kool t-owl* – a cold towel applied to the face after a shaving service in order to close the pores and prevent *infection*. It is prepared by running under cold running water and placing in mild refrigeration to cool.

Corkscrew twist – *kor-k-scroo tw-ist* – a method of *twisting* longer hair to create a spiral-like *twist*.

Corn row plaiting – *kor-n ro pla-ting* – a *plaiting* technique working along channels of hair, using three subsections of hair. Hair is woven either under or over to produce tight plaits that sit on the scalp. Also called 'cane row' plaiting. See also *braid*.

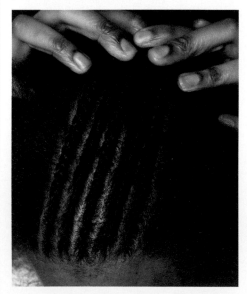

Corn row plaiting

Corrective relaxing – *kor-ek-tiv ru-lax-ing* – the process of *relaxing* hair, performed when hair which has been previously chemically relaxed has produced an uneven result.

Cortex – *kor-tex* – a major component of the *hair shaft* which provides strength and *elasticity* to the hair. It is made up of bundles of fibres. *Melanin* and *pheomelanin* are found here. In European hair the cortex runs evenly through the hair shaft; in African Caribbean hair there are two types of cortex which make the hair curly and dense. The cortex is where all the changes take place during *perming*, *colouring*, *relaxing* and *bleaching*. The flatter the shape of the cortex the easier and quicker it is for chemicals on the hair to be processed. (See the cortex diagram on page 160.)

Cosmetic Products (Safety) Regulations 2004 – *koz-me-tik pro-duk-tz say-f-tee reg-yoo-lay-shunz* – these are regulations regarding:

- composition of products
- ingredient labelling
- product description
- product marketing.

These can be useful to identify ingredients to which some clients may be allergic.

Cost effective – *kos-t u-fek-tiv* – producing the best results for the costs allowed.

Cotton wool – *kot-tn wul* – raw cotton with its wax removed. In hairdressing it is supplied as a thin coiled roll. It is used around the hairline before applying *perm lotion* and *neutraliser* to absorb and stop chemicals dripping on to the skin or clothes and into the eyes.

Counterfeit – *kow-n-tur-fit* – a fake or forged imitation of something. It usually refers to money, but also applies to debit or credit cards, passports, or a person's identification. It is illegal to produce counterfeit money and it is an offence to pass it on to others.

Course of action – *k-ors ov ak-shun* – the normal order of progress or the method of carrying out a service.

Courteous – *kurt-ee-us* – being *polite* and respectful.

31

Cowlick – *kow-lik* – a particular *hair growth pattern* in which the hair grows strongly to one side of the forehead and may stick up. As for a **widow's peak**, this may affect the cutting of a fringe as the hair will separate and stick out on one side. Working with the hair growth pattern produces the best results.

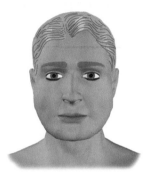

Cowlick hair growth pattern

Created locks – *kree-ayt-id l-ox* – locks formed by *intertwining* hair. See also *locking*, *yarn locks*.

Credit card – *kre-dit kard* – a thin plastic card provided by a bank or building society that contains security information, such as a signature or personal identification number (PIN). It authorises the person named on it to charge purchases or services to his or her account.

Creeping oxidation – *kree-ping oxi-day-shun* – occurs when residues of chemicals are left in the hair (not rinsed out correctly) and the chemical reactions they produce carry on working. This can cause damage to the hair. See also *oxidation*.

Crimp – *krim-p* – a process, using **crimping irons**, which creates temporary corrugated shapes in the hair.

Crimping irons – *krim-ping iy-unz* – electrical *equipment* with corrugated heated plates which are used to *crimp* hair.

Cross-check – *kr-os ch-ek* – to examine different sections of hair at the same time. This is done to ensure that the hair style is *balanced*, for example, checking that the *length* or layers of hair after *cutting* are even.

Cross-infection – *kr-os in-fek-shun* – the transfer of a *disease* or an *infection* from one person to another.

Cross-reference – *kr-os ref-ur-uns* – refer to a variety of written sources or texts on the same topic, especially when collating *evidence* for a project or task.

Crown – *kr-ow-n* – the top, most rounded part of the head shape.

Curl – *kur-l* – hair in the shape of a curve, spiral or coil. See also *curling*.

Curling – *kur-l-ing* – a technique used to form **curls**, usually in medium to longer length hair. It involves winding a mesh of wet hair around a circular tool (e.g. a brush or a roller), the stylist's fingers, or electrical **equipment** (e.g. **curling tongs**, or a hot brush) and adding heat. The **hydrogen bonds** in the hair take on the new shape.

Curling tongs – *kur-l-ing t-ong-z* – heated equipment used to temporarily curl hair. Hair is wound around the barrel of the tongs, and the heat penetrates the mesh of hair, effectively 'baking' the hair into taking on the shape of the barrel. The tongs are removed and the hair is allowed to cool to set the **curl** in place before **dressing out**. This produces small tight curls if used on short hair and spiral curls if used on longer lengths of hair. Also known as curling irons.

Custom blended hair – *kus-tum blen-did hayr* – **added hair** that is blended to the specific order of the client. After the client's hair colour is analysed, the added hair or hair extensions are blended to match the client's hair colour.

Customer services – *kus-tu-mur sur-vis-ez* – services for a particular business which meet the needs of clients. Good communication skills, an understanding of the market, the types of products required, awareness of the trends within the business, **client rights** and the legal requirements of the salon are all factors to consider when providing these services.

Cut-throat razor – *kut-th-rowt ray-zr* – a razor made of sharp steel that has either a fixed blade, which will require sharpening at regular intervals, or a *continued...*

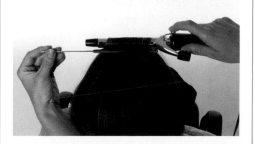

Using curling tongs

detachable blade, which is disposable. It has a hinged handle that pivots open when the blade needs to be used, and then can be closed back to protect the blade when not in use. Sometimes called *open blade razor*.

Cuticle – *kyoo-ti-kul* – the outermost layer of the *hair shaft*, made up of overlapping scales. When cuticle scales lie flat, the hair will appear shiny and healthy. Damaged cuticle scales lift away, making the hair feel rough and appear dull. The number of layers of scales depends on the hair type: coarse hair will have more cuticle layers, making it more resistant to chemical processes such as *perming*. If the cuticle is damaged by harsh treatments, chemicals or over-exposure to sunlight, hair will become *porous* and feel rough. (See the hair follicle diagram on page 159.)

Cutting – *kut-ing* – removing hair from the head, using a sharp tool such as *scissors* or a *razor*. See also *cutting comb*, *cutting guideline*.

Cutting comb – *kut-ing ko-m* – a comb used for sectioning and combing hair when *cutting*. It comes in a variety of sizes, with some being more flexible than others, for example, those used for cutting close to the nape or ears during *scissor-over-comb* work. Traditionally, longer or bigger combs are used for *barbering*.

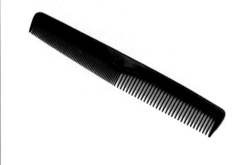

A cutting comb

Cutting guideline – *kut-ing giy-d-lyn* – a guide that is followed throughout a haircut to ensure accuracy. The first section cut becomes the guideline which is used for each subsequent section that is cut. This ensures evenness throughout the haircut and makes the *length* of each section more accurate. It is important to use a guideline for *cutting* hair, rather than using guesswork.

Dandruff – *dan-druf* – excessive production and shedding of the cells of the *epidermis* which lie on the scalp and in the hair, causing itchiness, redness and soreness due to scratching. Specialist *shampoos* and *conditioners* containing zinc pyrithione or selenium sulphide can be used; however, if the condition is severe, the client should be referred to a *trichologist*.

Data Protection Act 1998 – *day-ta pru-tek-shun akt* – this Act affects businesses using computer or paper-based systems for holding personal details of clients and staff. It states (among other points) that:

- information must be kept securely
- information must be accurate and relevant to the needs of the business
- businesses must comply with individuals' requests for information that is held on them.

Debit card – *deb-it kard* – a thin plastic card provided by a bank or building society that contains security information, such as a signature or personal identification number (PIN). It allows the person named on it to use it to pay for goods and services, if there are available funds in the account. See also *credit card*.

Defect – *dee-f-ekt* – a fault, usually found in goods. Defective *products* cannot be sold to a client, and the client has the right to return the product and receive a refund. See also *Sale of Goods Act 1979*.

Delivery – *du-liv-ur-ee* – 1. the distribution or supply of a *service* or *product*. All deliveries are treated in the same way: the *stock* arrives with a delivery note stating the contents of the delivery; the items are checked to ensure nothing is damaged; the delivery note is checked against the order to ensure it is has been filled correctly and there are no missing items; the delivery is then safely stored until required. 2. the manner in which a speech is given, for example, when delivering a training seminar.

Demonstrate – *de-mon-st-ray-t* – to *describe*, *explain* or *illustrate* by using practical examples or experiments.

Demonstration – *de-mon-st-ray-shun* – publicly showcasing the work, or promoting the **products**, of a salon. It can also refer to a situation in a classroom environment in which techniques are shown and explained by a teacher or lecturer.

Denman brush – *den-mun br-ush* – a brush with rigid plastic bristles, made by a company called Denman, used for **smoothing** and **straightening** hair.

Density – *den-sit-ee* – the amount of hair per square centimetre on the head.

Depth – *dep-th* – the lightness or darkness of a client's existing hair colour. It can be determined by matching up the hair colour with the column of colours that usually run down the right-hand side of a colour chart: 1 = black; 2 = dark brown; 3 = medium brown; 4 = light brown; 5 = lightest brown; 6 = dark blonde; 7 = medium blonde; 8 = light blonde; 9 = very light blonde; 10 = lightest blonde. Also known as **base colour**.

Dermal papilla – *dur-mul pu-pil-a* – (plural **papillae** – *pu-pil-iy*) – found in the **papillary layer** of the **dermis**. It is pear shaped and contains a rich blood supply through the capillary loops at its base, which in turn nourish the **follicle**. The papilla divides into two parts – the lower part contains unstructured cells which multiply rapidly. They change into specific hair cells only when they are pushed through the papilla towards the top. See also **dermis**, **mitosis**. (See the structure of the skin diagram and the hair follicle diagram on page 159.)

Dermatitis – *der-ma-tiyt-us* – **inflammation** or **allergy** of the skin. Usually affecting the hands of hairdressers, it causes the hands and fingers to crack and bleed due to constantly being wet and coming into contact with certain chemicals. Drying hands thoroughly after shampooing, using a good **barrier cream** and always wearing gloves when touching chemicals will help to avoid this. Sometimes called **contact dermatitis**.

Dermatologist – *der-ma-tol-o-jist* – a specialist who diagnoses (identifies) and treats skin disorders.

Dermis – *der-mis* – the layer of skin found between the **epidermis**

and the *subcutaneous layer*. It has fewer cells than the epidermis but more connective tissue for supporting the skin. It divides into the papillary layer and the reticular layer. The papillary layer is uppermost, and contains the nerve endings, blood supply, arrector pili muscle and lymph vessels. The reticular layer is the deepest of the skin's layers and is classed as connective tissue, made up of collagen and elastin fibres that give the skin structure and strength. (See the structure of the skin diagram on page 159.)

Describe – *des-criy-b* – to give an account of something by giving details of its characteristics.

Design – *du-ziyn* – to invent or plan something, for example, a new hairstyle.

Desired look – *du-ziyr-d luk* – a specific look requested by a client, often seen in a hairstyle magazine.

De-tangling – *dee-tang-ling* – the process of combing the hair from the points (ends of the hair) to the roots, to avoid knotting the hair and causing the client discomfort.

Developer – *du-vel-o-pur* – a solution of **hydrogen peroxide** used during a **colouring** service. Depending on how strong it is, it will soften and swell the **cuticle** slightly to allow the colouring **product** to **penetrate** better.

Development target – *du-vel-op-mnt tar-git* – an aim or a goal; something to strive towards. It can be personal, or one for all staff to achieve, such as aiming to sell a particular range of **products** or **services** over a period of time. It should be set within an achievable time scale to avoid staff feeling demoralised. See also **targets**.

Development test curl – *du-vel-op-mnt test kur-l* – a test carried out on the hair during the **perming** process to check whether the desired development of the **curl** has been reached.

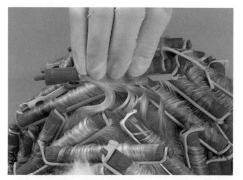

A development test curl

Diamond face shape – *diy-mund fay-s shay-p* – the **head and face shape** determined by a narrow bone structure of the forehead with wide cheekbones tapering to a narrow chin. The ideal hairstyle for this shape is one which minimises the width across the cheekbones. A central *fringe* should be worn with hair full below the cheeks but flat at the cheekbone line. (See head and face shapes on page 161.)

Different needs – *dif-r-unt nee-dz* – differing requirements, especially those of clients. It is illegal to discriminate against clients on grounds of disability, race, ethnicity or sex. See also *client needs*, *Disability Discrimination Act 1992, 1995 and 2005*, *Race Relations Act 2000*.

Diffuse alopecia – *dif-yoos alo-pee-sha* – a gradual loss of hair and thinning. Often appearing in women, it is thought to be due to changing *hormone* levels which have a direct affect on *hair follicles*. Pregnancy, the contraceptive pill and the menopause can all contribute to this type of hair loss. It can also be a symptom of some illnesses, such as a thyroid problem or iron deficiency, so the client should be referred to a **General Practitioner**.

Diffuser – *dif-yooz-ur* – a large plastic attachment, often with prongs, that fits on to a **hairdryer**. It distributes heat so that natural hair movement and curl are encouraged as the hair is dried. The end is placed directly on to the hair where the hair is worked around the fingers in a circular fashion. Being large and open it spreads the heat over a wider section of hair, allowing the hair to be dried slowly and increasing the amount of curl present. See also **finger dry**.

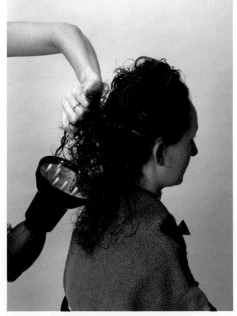

Using a diffuser

Diphtheria – *dif-thea-ree-ur* – a highly *contagious* bacterial *infection*. It is a notifiable *disease*, which means it must be reported to the Public Health Authorities by law. It causes a thick grey *membrane* to appear in patches on the skin, which bleeds on removal. The toxins (poisons) from the disease can attack the heart and nerves causing irreparable damage.

Directional perm winding – *diy-rek-shun-ul purm wiyn-ding* – a *directional winding* technique using *perm rods*.

Directional winding – *diy-rek-shun-ul wiyn-ding* – winding *rollers* or *perm rods* into the hair in a specific direction, similar to the way the client will wear the finished hairstyle.

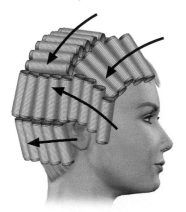

Directional winding

Direct observation – *diy-rekt obs-ur-vay-shun* – the process of directly observing, for example, an *assessor* viewing an *S/NVQ* candidate carrying out tasks which relate to *unit* standards. At times, only parts of a *service* will be observed: for example, when a candidate wishes to be observed for the hair *analysis* and shampooing part of a treatment, but is not yet confident in *cutting* skills. See also *assessment*.

Disability Discrimination Acts 1992, 1995 and 2005 – *dis-u-bil-it-ee dis-krim-in-ay-shun akts* – an Act which states that a person must not discriminate against a person with any disability. In a salon every person has a duty to promote equal opportunities for disabled persons as well as those who are not disabled.

Discount – *dis-k-ow-nt* – money off, or a reduction or mark down in price. See also *calculate*.

Discrepancy – *dis-krep-un-see* – (plural **discrepancies** – *dis-krep-un-seez*) – a difference between items or a disagreement between people's understanding of something.

Discussion – *dis-ku-shun* – a conversation, such as a *consultation* to determine **client needs**.

Disease – *diz-eez* – a *disorder* which can be severe or mild. Some forms are **contagious** – spread by direct contact, through touching; others are **infectious** – spread by inhaling contaminated droplets or through touching an infected object (towels, gowns, gloves, etc). (See infectious diseases of the skin and scalp on pages 162–163.)

Disorder – *dis-or-dur* – a disturbance or abnormality of physical or mental health or function.

Display – *dis-play* – show something in order to draw attention to it, for example, **products** in a salon's **reception** area.

Disposable blade razor – *dis-poz-ubul b-layd ray-zr* – a sharp blade used in **razoring**, designed to be disposable (thrown away). Because it is easy to replace, it is a popular choice for **health and safety** reasons. Also called **safety razor**.

Disposable cape – *dis-poz-ubul kay-p* – a large, plastic cape tied around the client's shoulders to protect the clothes, which is later thrown away.

Disulphide bond – *diy-sul-fiyd bon-d* – two sulphur **atoms** bonded together, found within the **cortex** region of the hair. Forming part of the protein of the hair (**keratin**) these bonds help to maintain the hair's **elasticity**. Being strong, they can only be broken by the addition of a chemical such as **perm lotion**.

Divide – *di-viyd* – to separate into parts. See also **parting**.

Documentary evidence – *dok-yoo-men-t-aree ev-i-dens* – a factual record of work kept and stored in a logical format to provide information of facts and **evidence**. For an **S/NVQ** candidate, it is used to support practical **assessments**. For example, copies of minutes of meetings or discussions can sometimes be the only source of proof; consultation sheets and worksheets, and witness statements signed and dated, are also excellent sources of evidence.

Documentation – *dok-yoo-men-tay-shun* – any paperwork or record of work found in a **workplace**, such as minutes of a meeting, delivery notes, personal certificates, a staff notice or target settings.

Double base – *dub-l bay-s* – twice as much **base colour**, represented on a colour chart by the same number appearing twice (for example, 66 or 55). Used on **white hair** or **resistant hair**, it ensures an intense and better coverage of the base colour: the base shade acts as an 'undercoat', and if the hair is resistant (has closed **cuticles** or lots of cuticle scales), the double base will provide better coverage on the hair, thereby achieving the **target colour**.

Double perm winding – *dub-l purm wiyn-ding* – a technique in which a **perm rod** is wound normally to mid-length, another rod placed against the first rod, then both rods wound together to the root area. This produces a tighter **curl** at the ends of the hair, with a looser curl at mid-length and at the roots. Also called double wind.

Dreadlocks – *dred-lox* – hairstyle whereby (long) hair is twisted or tightly curled, often worn by followers of the African Caribbean Rastafarian cult. See also **locking**.

Dressing cream – *d-res-ing kreem* – a **finishing product** used at the end of the **styling** process to define the finished continued...

Double crown – *dub-l kr-ow-n* – the **hair growth pattern** consisting of two swirls of hair on the crown of the head, growing clockwise around each centre. Hair should not be cut too short in this area as it will stick up; it is best to work with the direction of the growth.

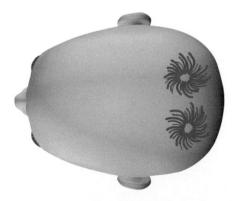

Double crown hair growth

style and add texture. Excess amounts make the hair greasy and lank.

Dressing out – *d-res-ing ow-t* – removing **roller** marks from the hair created during a **setting** process then **backcombing** or teasing the hair into place to create lift and **volume**.

Dressing-out comb – *d-res-ing-ow-t ko-m* – a rigid, plastic comb sometimes having metal prongs on one end to aid finer dressing-out techniques. A comb with small teeth is used when stiff **backcombing** is required to produce a tighter effect. The prongs of the comb are used when only a small amount of teasing is needed.

Dry – *driy* – lacking in moisture. To improve general health of hair and scalp, nourishing products, such as coconut oil or almond oil shampoo, may need to be applied.

Dry setting – *driy set-ing* – a **setting** method whereby **setting aids**, such as thermal lotions and **sprays**, are placed directly on the hair without firstly shampooing the hair. This does not break down the **hydrogen bonds** so the hair must be 'baked' into its new shape around **rollers**. It is a quick method used to support hair-up styles rather than having to carry out a full setting process. See also **wet setting**.

Dual action perm – *dyoo-ul ak-shun purm* – a **perming** process which uses specific chemicals applied twice to perm African Caribbean hair. It is kinder to hair than a **single action perm**.

Duty holder – *dyoo-tee hold-ur* – the person who takes full **responsibility** for all aspects of **health and safety**, **risk assessment** and understands the full legal requirements within the workplace. Members of a salon may rotate in shifts to be the duty holder. The duty holder is often also the first aider.

Eczema – *ek-z-mur* – a non-infectious skin condition, which is associated with **allergic reactions** and being sensitive to drugs or chemicals. It can be mild or severe but is always itchy. Scratching can cause **infection**, often a fungal infection with **papules** and **pustules** which may give off a discharge and later become scaly and crusted. It responds well to cream application of hydrocortisone (a steroid) and emollient creams which moisturise, soothe and soften the skin. It is not uncommon for hairdressers to develop the condition on the hands because of contact with **shampoos**, **conditioners** and chemicals: **gloves** and **barrier creams** are very effective in preventing the skin from becoming more irritated. If a fungal infection is present, the condition responds very well to **antibiotics**.

Effective – *u-fek-tiv* – useful, of value, such as making good use of time and resources, or the successful management of staff.

Effleurage massage – *ef-lur-aj mas-arj* – slow, smooth, stroking massage movements done with the palms of the hands during shampooing and conditioning. It is done in order to apply **products** or to relax the client.

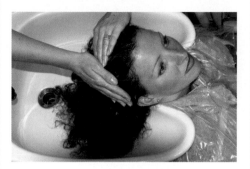
Effleurage

Elasticity – *ee-las-tis-it-ee* – the ability of something to return to its normal shape after being stretched. In hair, the **condition** or strength of the **cortex** determines this ability. Hair with good elasticity will stretch and recoil to its original **length** without becoming damaged, whilst hair in poor condition will over stretch and may even break off if put under pressure.

Elasticity test – *ee-las-tis-it-ee test* – a test done on hair to check if there is any internal damage to the **hair shaft**, carried out before **colouring**, **perming**, **corrective relaxing**, heat **styling** and general styling. It is done by lifting a few strands of hair away from continued...

the scalp and pulling them gently between the thumb and fingers to test their *elasticity*. When stretched it should return to its normal *length*. If the hair does not spring back to its original shape and length, it indicates there is internal damage and, if treated, the hair will over stretch and may break off.

Electricity at Work Regulations 1989 – *u-lek-tri-sit-ee at wurk reg-yoo-lay-shunz* – this Act states that all electrical equipment must be regularly checked for electrical safety by a competent person.

Electronic – *e-lek-tron-ik* – operated electrically, such as machinery or a computer.

Electronic authorisation – *e-lek-tron-ik or-th-riy-zay-shun* – approval made *electronically*. It may be necessary to phone the bank or clearing house for an *authorisation* code to enable an electronic payment to go ahead. This does not automatically mean that the client has gone over their spending limit – often banks do random security checks for quality control. See also *debit* and *credit card*.

Elements – *el-u-ments* – the smaller parts of a hairdressing

S/NVQ unit. In the unit overview they may be referred to as outcomes. Each one describes a particular task that will provide *evidence*.

Emergency – *u-mur-jen-see* – an occurrence, usually of danger, which requires immediate action.

Emerging look – *u-mur-jing luk* – a commercial look which is the forerunner of fashion. Next season's looks are generally set by fashion houses during catwalk shows.

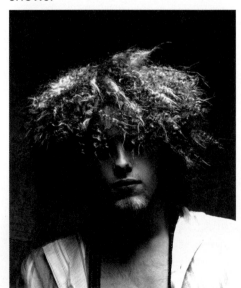

An emerging look

Employee – *em-ploy-ee* – a person who is hired to work for a person or company in return for payment.

Employer – *em-ploy-ur* – a person or company who gives work to *employees* and pays them.

Employers' Liability (Compulsory Insurance) Act 1969 – *em-ploy-urz liy-u-bi-litee kom-pul-sor-ee in-syoor-uns akt* – this Act states that employers and self-employed persons must hold *liability insurance* to insure them against any liability for body injury, illness or disease to their employees arising out of their employment.

End paper – *end pay-pur* – a small paper applied to the ends of hair before winding the hair onto a *perm rod*. This stops the ends of the hair becoming buckled.

Enhance – *en-harn-s* – to make more valuable or attractive. For example, a finished hairstyle should *complement* the client's positive features.

Enhance salon image – *en-harn-s sal-on im-ij* – to positively increase the salon's reputation. Advertising, promotions and special offers may be used to do this.

Enquiry – *in-kwiyr-ee* – a *question*, request for information, or a query. It is important that it is answered *professionally*, or is passed on to someone who is more able to help.

Environmental damage – *en-vy-ron-ment-ul dam-ij* – hair damaged by *environmental factors*, such as over-exposure to the sun, or pollution.

Environmental factors – *en-vy-ron-ment-ul fakt-urs* – features that are within and outside one's surroundings. In a salon environment, potential *hazards* or *high risk* factors to consider are chemicals which are flammable (easily set on fire), running water, heated *equipment* and use of electricity.

Epidermis – *ep-i-dur-mis* – the outermost layer of the skin, above the *dermis*, consisting of five layers (from the bottom): *basal layer, prickle cell layer, granular layer, clear layer, horny layer*. It contains no blood vessels and is made up of special cells which change shape according continued...

to their role within the skin. As the cells change they move up through the layers and become filled with **keratin**. They eventually reach the horny layer where the dead skin cells are sloughed off (fall away). (See the structure of the skin diagram on page 159.)

Epilepsy – ep-il-ep-see – a nervous **disorder**, sometimes due to brain damage, which causes fits. This medical problem is a **contraindication** to some scalp massage techniques, for example, the use of **high frequency** treatments.

Equal opportunities – ee-kwul op-ur-tyoon-it-eez – the assurance that every person will have the same chances in life, regardless of their age, gender, ethnic group, marital status. See also **Disability Discrimination Act 1992, 1995 and 2005** and **Race Relations Act 2000**.

Equipment – u-kwip-mnt – tools and other items, both fixed and mobile, that are used to carry out **services**. Some examples in a hairdressing salon include **backwash basins, hairdryers, scissors**, mirrors and **perm rods**.

Erythema – er-i-thee-mur – a redness of the skin, due to an accumulation of **blood** in the **capillaries** of the skin. Massage, heat, **inflammation** or an **allergy** often cause this condition. It may also be present at the site of an infection. Reddening of the skin or scalp may be a **contraindication** to a service, so it is important to avoid aggravating or over-stimulating the area.

Essential knowledge and understanding (EKU) – u-sen-shul no-lij nd un-dur-stan-ding – vital information of which a person or an **S/NVQ** candidate needs to show understanding. It is the background theory that supports a candidate's practical treatments. Also called **knowledge evidence**. See also **assessment**.

Estimated price – es-ti-may-td priy-s – a guide or educated guess of the cost of something, such as the price of a **service** or **product**. It should be within a small margin for error.

Ethical standards – eth-i-kul stand-urds – principles or **ethics** outlining moral **behaviour**. **Professional** ethics dictate how to behave, treat clients and conduct business in a proper way. See also *Code of Practice*.

Ethics – *eth-iks* – a set of values or principles, especially in relation to a particular field. See also *Code of Practice*.

Ethos – *ee-th-os* – an outlook or philosophy. If the work ethos of staff is good, it will generate a positive salon atmosphere for both staff and customers.

Eumelanin – *yoo-mel-a-nin* – natural black/brown colour pigments which produce *cool tones* in hair. See also *melanin*.

Evaluate – *e-val-yoo-ayt* – to judge the worth of something or a situation. Methods include verbal feedback and using questionnaires to gain written feedback from *colleagues* or an external group of people.

Evaluation – *e-val-yoo-ay-shun* – the judgement of something or a situation, which can be done informally, such as during discussion, or, formally, in a written report. For example, in a staff meeting, the effects of changing an aspect of customer service can be evaluated.

Evidence – *ev-i-duns* – proof. In hairdressing, *S/NVQ* candidates use this to show they have met the *assessment* criteria and have gained the level of competency as stated in a *unit*. See also *assessment*.

Excessive tension – *ex-ses-iv ten-shun* – the application of too much force when stretching something. For example, if too much tension is applied when attaching *hair extensions* the consequences can be *traction alopecia* or hair loss.

Excess moisture – *ex-ses moy-s-chur* – too much water present. If hair is too wet to carry out the next *service*, moisture must be removed by drying it with a towel or a *hairdryer*.

Excrete – *ex-kreet* – to eliminate waste products from the body, such as salts from *sweat glands* in the skin.

Exfoliation – *ex-fol-iy-ay-shun* – the removal of dead *epidermal* skin cells. This is a natural process which helps new cells to come through the skin, but can be speeded up by the use of a loofah, massage or the *continued...*

application of creams with synthetic beads in them, which exfoliate the top layers of the epidermis. This keeps the skin looking fresh, by avoiding a *build-up* of dead skin cells and preventing *in-growing hair* from developing. (See the structure of the skin diagram on page 159.)

Existing colour – *ex-sist-ing kul-ur* – colour that is already present. For example, this may be a client's natural hair colour or an artificial colour from a previous *colouring* treatment.

Explain – *ex-play-n* – to give an account of something in a clear way so that it can be easily understood by someone else.

Explanation – *ex-plan-ay-shun* – a description that makes something clear.

External Verification – *ex-tur-nul veri-fi-kay-shun* – a system put in place by a body or organisation which ensures that the standards and *assessment* systems of a course are being maintained nationally. An *External Verifier* (EV) is the main link between an *Awarding Body* and an assessment centre or college.

External Verifier – *ex-tur-nul veri-fiy-ur* – a person (often called an EV) appointed by an *External Verification* body to ensure that national standards in a subject area are being met. He or she has appropriate qualifications and vocational experience and knowledge and normally visits a centre or college twice a year. The EV provides feedback to the *Awarding Body* on the standards observed and also supports the college or centre for future development of *qualifications* or any resources needed.

Face shape – *fay-s shay-p* – see *head and face shape*.

Facial hair outline – *fay-sh-l hayr owt-l-yn* – the shape of facial hair left on the face once unwanted hair is removed from outside the beard, *moustache* or *sideburns*. It is important to wet and apply lather only to the areas where hair is to be removed. The hair is removed by holding the skin taut and shaving in the direction of the hair growth.

Facial piercing – *fay-sh-l peer-s-ing* – jewellery on the face, usually placed through holes in the nose, lip or eyebrows. They need to be moved prior to *barbering* to prevent injury to the client.

Factor – *fak-tur* – a detail or *feature* that determines the result of something. Aspects of a *service* on a client should be noted on the *client record*, for example, if the client had a poor reaction to a *colouring* or perm test or to the actual service, as it may limit the services or choice of *products* that can be offered to the client in the future. It is also worth noting a client's personal preference for a particular brand or make of colour.

Fading – *fay-ding* – creating a hairline without bold or harsh edges. It is usually carried out on African Caribbean hair using *scissor-over-comb*, *clipper-over-comb* or *freehand* techniques.

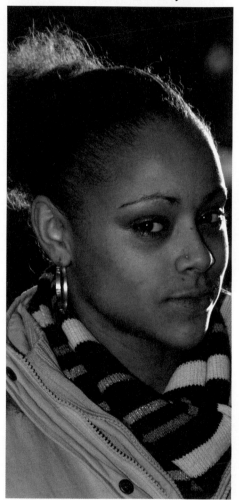
Faded hairline

49

Fashion trend – *fa-shun tr-end* – a popular or high profile hairstyle. Often a client may want to copy a particular look of a celebrity, or wish to have an up-dated hairstyle with a more modern look. However, the style should always be adapted to suit the *client's features* and hair type. See also *emerging look*.

Fatigue – *fat-ee-g* – tiredness as a result of carrying out an activity.

Feature – *fee-chur* – a quality or characteristic of something. For example, a hairstyle should always *complement* the *client's features*, or when *selling* a *product*, a *stylist* should understand the benefits of the product. See also *benefits of products*.

Feedback – *feed bak* – comments or advice on an event or action that has taken place, for example, those given by an assessor on the performance of an *S/NVQ* candidate.

Finger dry – *fin-gur driy* – a way of drying hair by using the hands and fingers to encourage movement and curl in the hair. It can also be used to create short, spiky, textured styles. See also *diffuser*, *scrunch dry*.

Finger waving – *fin-gur way-ving* – a *styling* technique that works with the natural movement in the hair to form flat waves or deep crests and troughs in the hair. The end result creates an 's' shape formation. This technique will not produce any *root lift* in the hair, so the use of strong *styling* products is required. The most suitable type of hair for using this technique is on medium to fine textured hair of a reasonable *length* that has some natural movement.

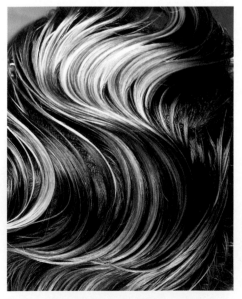

The end result of finger waving

Finishing product – *fin-ish-ing pro-duk-t* – a *product* which can be used on wet or dry hair to help achieve the finished result, such as *dressing cream*, *oils*, *sprays*, *wax* and *gel*.

Fire Precautions (Workplace) Regulations 1997 – *fiy-r pre-kor-shunz wurk-play-s reg-yoo-lay-shunz* – this Act states that business owners must adequately assess fire risks associated with their work activities and decide what needs to be done to control the risks.

Fish hooks – *fish huks* – hair ends that have become buckled or bent during *winding*. They need to be removed by *cutting*.

Fishtail plait – *fish-tay-l plat* – a style in which all hair is incorporated into a *plait* which starts at the forehead and finishes at the *nape*.

Fixing (stage) – *fix-ing stay-j* – a stage in the *perming* process, involving *neutralising* which removes hydrogen from the *cortex* of the hair by adding oxygen (see *oxidation*). This process joins together sulphur bonds to re-form *disulphide*

bonds in a new position, which permanently fixes the *curl*.

Flat barrel curl – *flat ba-rel kur-l* – a *curl* that lies flat on the head with an open middle. It is even from roots to points (ends of hair). See also *pin curling*.

Flat brush – *flat br-ush* – sometimes referred to as a paddle brush, it can have a solid flat back or an open back to allow the *airflow* to pass through it. This creates movement in the hair and allows the hair to dry more quickly.

Float – *flow-t* – the sum of money left in a till at the end of the day to be given as change to clients on the next working day. It is deducted from the daily *takings* and not counted when tallying up the accounts.

Flow – *flo* – the rate of movement, for example, how fast or slow water comes out of a tap.

Foils – *foy-lz* – thin, metal sheets, similar to cooking foil, that keep heat within a packet to aid the development of a *colouring* process. They come on a roll and can be cut to suit the hair *continued...*

51

length and folded into neat packets that can be placed anywhere on the head.

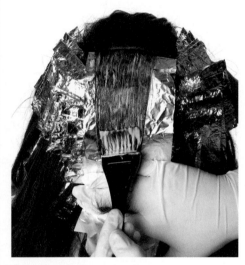

Using foils during colouring

Folliculitis – *fo-lik-yoo-liy-tus* – inflammation of the *hair follicles*. (See the hair follicle diagram on page 159 and infectious diseases of the skin and scalp on pages 162–163.)

Foreseeable problem – *for-see-a-bul prob-lum* – a problem which is able to be predicted. A contingency plan can be made to avoid this type of problem occurring. For example, when planning for a hair show, it is important for stand-in models to practise, in case a model becomes ill before the show.

Fraud – *fr-or-d* – cheating or deception, usually to gain financial rewards. See also *counterfeit*.

Fraudulent use of card – *fr-or-dyoo-lnt yoos ov kar-d* – criminal use of a credit or debit card. See also *counterfeit*.

Freehand – *free-han-d* – *cutting* the hair without holding it with tension. The hair is combed into place and then cut freehand. Commonly used for cutting *fringes* and around the *nape* area and ears.

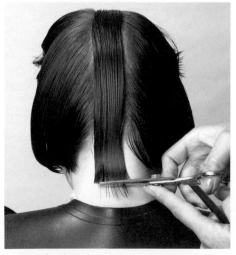

Cutting freehand

French plait – *fren-ch plat* – see *scalp plait*.

French pleat – *fren-ch plee-t* – see *vertical roll*.

Friction massage – *frik-shun mas-arj* – light, quick massage movements using the pads of the fingers which gently stimulates the scalp during shampooing.

Fringe – *frin-j* – the part of the hair that covers the forehead. The different types include: straight and heavy, *texturised*, asymmetric (longer on one side than the other), very short, or long, which can cover one or both eyes.

Frizziness – *fri-z-ee-nus* – a mass of hair with small, tight *curls* which knots easily. This can be a sign of hair damage caused by over-processing of *perm lotion* or *neutralising* lotion.

Front wash basin – *frunt wosh bays-n* – a basin which is used for shampooing the hair of a client who has back or neck problems, or a client, such as a child, who is too small to lean back into a *backwash basin*. After putting a gown on the client, a towel is placed around the front as well as around the shoulders. The client is then given a towel to protect the eyes and face before leaning forward into the basin.

Frosting – *fros-ting* – a *colouring* technique used on short, spiky hair. A lightening *product* is usually painted on to cling film or a *wrap* that is brushed along the top of the hair so the ends are coated with the product. This produces a natural colour effect. Also called **shoe shining**.

Full facial hair – *f-ul fay-sh-l hayr* – a term that refers to both the beard and moustache on the face, which is sometimes called the 'full set'.

Full head – *f-ul hed* – all the hair. For example, a full head colour means all the hair is coloured (see *full head application*), and full head *plaits* implies all the hair is plaited.

Full head application – *f-ul hed ap-li-kay-shun* – the application of colour to all the hair on the head. If a client has not had their hair coloured before this is classed as *virgin hair*, and the colour should be applied to the mid-lengths, then the ends and finally the roots. This *continued...*

allows for **body heat**, **porous** hair etc.

Fungus – *fun-gus* – (plural **fungi** – *fun-g-ee*) – a uni- or multi-cellular organism. See also *infection*.

Fungal infection – *fun-gul in-fek-shun* – an *infection* caused by a **fungus**, for example **ringworm**. (See infectious diseases of the skin and scalp on pages 162–163.)

Fuse – *f-yooz* – to combine or join together. For example, a method of joining **hair extensions** to natural hair is by melting a substance to fix them securely.

Future services – *fyoo-chur sur-vis-ez* – services the client may want in the coming weeks or months. Testing may need to be done before carrying these out, which should be listed on the **client record**. See also **necessary tests**.

Gel – *j-el* – a **product** used for **styling** or finishing hair, available in tubs, tubes and in spray form. Stronger than **mousse** or other lotions, it is used for sculpting wet hair. It is ideal for short, thick, dense hair, **texturised** or spiky styles that require a strong hold. It is not suitable for fine hair as its heaviness may weigh the hair down. It also protects the hair from **atmospheric moisture**. The amount of product to be applied depends on the desired style: for a slicked back look, a large amount is needed; for a slight amount of lift at the root area the product needs to be used sparingly.

General Practitioner (GP) – *jen-rul prak-tish-un-ur* – a medical doctor who diagnoses (identifies) illnesses and **diseases** and treats patients. A GP will refer a patient on to a specialist within a particular field of medicine, if specialised testing or treatment is required.

General Product Safety Regulations 1994 – *jen-rul pro-duk-t say-f-tee reg-yoo-lay-shunz* – these regulations deal with product safety and, in part, replace the **Consumer Protection Act**. It is the responsibility of all businesses to ensure that their products are safe.

Germinal matrix – *jer-min-ul may-t-rix* – the section of the skin where cells reproduce to form the **hair shaft** within the **hair bulb**. (See the structure of the skin diagram on page 159.)

Gland – *glan-d* – an organ in the body that produces and secretes (releases) chemical substances, such as **sebum** from the **sebaceous** glands in the skin.

Gloves – *glu-vz* – protective covering for hands. They are used during chemical treatments to avoid staining and irritating the skin which can lead to conditions such as **dermatitis**.

Good practice – *gud pr-ak-tis* – as an individual, behaving **professionally** and responsibly at all times with both colleagues and clients; as a salon, having an **equal opportunities** policy in place as well as correct procedures for promoting health and safety within the **workplace**.

Gown – *gow-n* – a large cape wrapped around the *continued…*

client's clothes to protect them during a hairdressing **service**.

Grades – *gr-aydz* – see **clipper attachments**.

Graduating – *grad-yoo-ayt-ing* – **cutting** the hair at different **lengths** and blending them together, for example, blending long layers into shorter layers or short layers into longer layers. The effect produced is called blended **layering**. See also **short graduation** and **long graduation**.

Granular layer – *gran-yoo-lur lay-ur* – the third layer of the **epidermis** of the skin found between the **clear layer** and the **prickle cell layer**. The cells within this layer begin to die: they are flatter and contain less fluid than the cells in the layer beneath them. (See the structure of the skin diagram on page 159.)

Greasy – *gree-see* – when referring to the hair or scalp, an excessive amount of natural **sebum** (grease) produced by the **sebaceous glands**. It can become worse through vigorous massage as this stimulates the glands to secrete more sebum. Specialist **shampoos** and **conditioners** will help to regulate the production of sebum, and a shampoo with lemon as an ingredient will help to remove excess grease.

Grievance – *gr-ee-v-uns* – a cause for complaint, such as a case of ill-treatment or unfairness, which can be experienced by either members of staff or a client. It is important to deal with complaints promptly, politely and in a **professional** manner. See also **grievance procedure** and **legislation** for **equal opportunities** and **disability discrimination**.

Grievance procedure – *gr-ee-v-uns pro-see-dyur* – a process set up to deal with a **grievance** in a correct and appropriate manner. All staff members in a salon should feel able to pursue this course of action without discrimination, if they have been treated unfairly.

Group assistance – *gr-oop us-ist-uns* – the cooperation or support of a team. For example, during a **promotional** evening to launch a new **product** range at a salon, all staff members may be required to help.

Guidance – *giy-duns* – *advice* or assistance on how to do something, or to help and support someone.

Guidelines – *giy-d-liy-nz* – *instructions* or principles. In a salon, rules should be established which fit within a legal framework. Displaying them or making them clear will help staff to follow the correct procedures. See also *good practice* and *Code of Practice*.

Hair – *hayr* – a number of thread-like fibres growing out of the skin. Each is made up a *hair bulb* which grows from the *dermis*, then extends as a *hair shaft* above the skin's surface. (See the structure of the skin diagram and the hair follicle diagram on page 159.) See also *dermis*.

Hair breaking – *hayr bray-k-ing* – hair snapping or separating due to being in poor *condition*. Causes include the results of poor colour application, *over-processing* of a *chemical service*, incorrect choice of *products* or the hair being in generally bad condition.

Hair bulb – *hayr bu-lb* – the section at the base of a hair from which the hair grows. It has two distinctive parts: the upper bulb and the *germinal matrix*. In the germinal matrix all the cells look the same, but in the upper bulb the hair starts to develop into its three layers: *medulla*, *cortex* and *cuticle*. (See the hair follicle diagram on page 159.) See also *dermal papilla* and *dermis*.

Hair characteristics – *hayr kar-ak-tur-is-tiks* – the *features* of hair such as its texture, *density*, strength and structure. Hair is classed as being fine, medium or coarse. It can also be curly or straight. This is thought to be influenced by the shape of the *hair follicle*, the rate of cell division (*mitosis*), *keratinisation*, as well as the client's ethnic origin. The shape of the follicle determines whether someone has straight, wavy or curly hair. Curly hair is largely produced in Black or African Caribbean skin, whilst Oriental or Asian skin tends to produce straight hair. Caucasian or European skins can produce either. (See the structure of the skin and the hair follicle diagram on page 159.)

Hair condition – *hayr kon-di-shun* – the degree of flatness and smoothness of the *cuticle* in the outer layer of the *hair shaft*. If the cuticle lies flat then light will reflect off it giving the hair a healthy, shiny appearance; if the

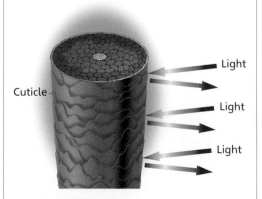

Cuticle

Light

Light

Light

Hair in good condition

cuticle is rough and bumpy the light will scatter in all directions making the hair look dull and damaged. By carrying out an *elasticity test* and a *porosity test* the inner and outer strength of the hair structure can be determined.

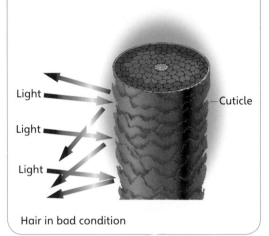

Hair in bad condition

Haircut – *hayr-kut* – the style in which a client's hair is cut.

Hair disorder – *hayr dis-or-dur* – a non-infectious condition of the hair which requires special consideration. As the requested *treatment* needs to be adapted for the *condition* of the client's hair, the client should be made aware of the limitations of the treatment in the initial *consultation*. See also *contraindication*.

Hairdressing and Beauty Industry Authority (HABIA) – *hayr-dres-ing nd byoo-tee in-dust-ree or-thor-it-ee* – a government-approved body which sets standards and addresses issues on hair, beauty, nails, spa therapy, *barbering* and African Caribbean hair. Its standards form the basis for all *qualifications* including *National Vocational Qualifications* (NVQs), *Scottish Vocational Qualifications* (SVQs) and Apprenticeships, as well as *Codes of Practice*. It also provides *guidance* on careers, business development, *legislation*, salon safety, *equal opportunities*, and is responsible to government on industry issues such as training and skills.

Hairdryer – *hayr-driy-ur* – a hand-held piece of electrical equipment used in a salon for drying hair.

Hair extension – *hayr ex-ten-shun* – a *length* of human or synthetic (man-made) hair which can be added to existing hair to increase *volume* and length to the hair.

Hair follicle – *hayr fol-i-kul* – the pocket below the surface of the skin in which a hair continued...

grows. (See the hair follicle diagram on page 159.)

Hair growth cycle – *hayr gro-w-th siy-kul* – the stages in the life cycle of hair, which are known as *anagen*, *catagen* and *telogen*. A single strand of hair does not grow continuously; *hair follicles* undergo alternate periods of activity, when the hair is growing. Hair, skin and nail growth is faster in the summer, slows down slightly in the winter and can be affected by ill health, drugs, poor nutrition, *hormone* fluctuation, such as during pregnancy, and when there is a poor *blood supply* to the area. As all the hairs do not grow at the same rate, the hair needs to be cut and shaped regularly to keep its style. (See the hair growth cycle diagram on page 160.)

Hair growth pattern – *hayr gro-w-th pat-urn* – an arrangement of the hair as it grows on the head. The direction in which the hair falls depends on the angle of the *follicle*. As little can be done to alter this, it is better to work with the hair direction, rather than against it. There are several types of patterns: *double crown*, *widow's peak*, *cowlick*, *nape whorl*. (See hair follicle diagram on page 159.)

Hair health – *hayr hel-th* – the physical **condition** of hair. The state of hair depends on the atmosphere and the seasons, the quality of nourishment it receives through diet, **hormonal** influences, effects of any medication taken, the amount of care given to it, and the type of **products** used on it. Head massage is good for promoting healthy hair as it stimulates hair growth by increasing the **blood supply** to the area.

Hair nerves – *hayr ner-vz* – the nerve supply to the hair. These nerves are attached to the **dermal papilla** in the **subcutaneous layer** of the skin. For example, if the hair is pulled, the client will feel a tugging of the skin. However, no pain will be felt by the client when the hair is cut, because there is no nerve supply to the **hair shaft** itself. (See the structure of the skin diagram on page 159.) See also *dermis*.

Hair shaft – *hayr sha-ft* – the part of the hair which is visible above the skin or scalp. It is mostly made up of dead cells and has no nerve supply (see *hair nerves*). Its structure consists of the **medulla** – the inner layer; the **cortex** – all chemical and physical processes take place here; the *cuticle* – the outer layer, made up of overlapping scales. (See the hair follicle diagram on page 159.)

Hair show – *hayr sho* – an event which gives hairdressers an opportunity to showcase their practical skills. This can involve *competition work* suitable for all levels of hairdressers or the chance to present the season's latest trends.

Hair spray – *hayr sp-ray* – see *sprays*.

Hairstyle – *hayr stiy-l* – the way in which a person's hair is styled.

Hair testing – *hayr tes-ting* – carrying out *analysis* on the hair and scalp to test suitability for a *service* or *product*. See also *necessary tests*.

Hair types – *hayr tiy-pz* – 1. varieties of hair. There are three categories: *lanugo hair* which develops on the baby in the womb from about the fifth month of pregnancy and disappears a few weeks after birth; *vellus hair* which is the soft, fine, downy hair, without *pigment*, that appears on all parts of the body except the palms of the hands and the soles of the feet; *terminal hair* which is strong, often coarse hair, most commonly found on the head, eyebrows, legs, underarms and pubic area. Its colour is determined by inherited family genes and it can be styled, cut or coloured quite easily. 2. relating to the three main hair types: European/Caucasian; African/Caribbean; Asian.

Hazard – *haz-ud* – something which is capable of causing harm or is dangerous, for example, a trailing cable or water spillage on the floor.

Hazardous substance – *haz-ud-us sub-stuns* – a substance which is a danger to people's health and safety. It needs to be stored, handled, used and disposed of carefully, using the correct methods outlined in the *manufacturer's instructions*.

Head and face shape – *hed nd fay-s shay-p* – the outline and contours of the head and face, determined by the underlying facial bones and the amount of fat in the underlying tissues. It is an important consideration when choosing a *hairstyle* for continued...

the client during a *consultation*, as the style needs to enhance the *client's features* rather than highlight possible flaws. For example, it would not be suitable to cut a straight fringe across a large flat forehead. (See head and face shapes on page 161.)

clean, tidy and free of waste. Also see *Health and Safety at Work Act 1974*.

Health and Safety at Work Act 1974 (HASWA) – *hel-th nd say-f-tee ut wurk akt* – an Act for securing the health, safety and

Head lice – *hed liys* – (pediculosis capitis) – small *parasites* which bite the scalp, suck blood from the host and cause itchiness. They are highly *contagious*, multiply rapidly and are commonly found behind the ears and at the hairline, although they can appear as an *infestation* over the whole head. (It is a myth that they appear only on dirty hair.) Although they cannot jump, the insects are spread through direct contact (head to head, especially in children) or through indirect contact (from brushes, combs etc.) and lay eggs (nits) on the hair shaft. The eggs cling to the shaft and cannot be removed by ordinary combing. Regular sectioning and combing with a nit comb from a pharmacy – for three weeks, to collect all the eggs in its life cycle – is one method of removal. (See infectious diseases of the skin and scalp on pages 162–163.)

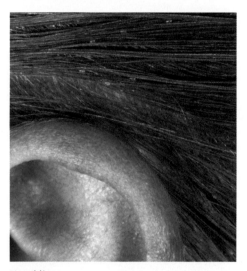

Head lice

Health and safety – *hel-th nd say-f-tee* – a term referring to practices in the *workplace* which ensure that *risks* and *hazards* to health and safety are reduced, for example, keeping work areas

welfare of persons at work, and for protecting others against risks to health or safety in connection with the activities of persons at work. There are many subsections covering:

- general duties of employers to their employees
- general duties of employees at work
- general duties of manufacturers regarding articles and substances for use at work
- possession and use of dangerous substances
- controlling certain offensive emissions into the atmosphere
- guidance for the employment medical advisory service
- building regulations.

Health and Safety Executive (HSE) – *hel-th nd say-f-tee ex-ek-yoo-tiv* – the Commission responsible for *health and safety* regulation in the United Kingdom. Its mission, along with local government, is to protect people's health and safety, by ensuring *risks* in the changing workplace are properly controlled.

Health and safety inspectors – *hel-th nd say-f-tee in-spek-tors* – people appointed by the *Health and Safety Executive* to ensure the standards outlined in the *Health and Safety at Work Act 1974* are being met in the *workplace*. They also investigate accidents and complaints, and promote understanding of what is required. Inspectors have the authority to enter a premises, if they feel a *risk* or *hazard* is present, and have the power to prosecute, should it be proven that a salon owner is not following all regulations.

Heart face shape – *hart fay-s shay-p* – the *head and face shape* determined by a wide forehead and the face tapering to a long jaw line. A suitable hairstyle for this shape is one which reduces the width across the forehead and emphasises the jaw line. (See head and face shapes on page 161.)

Heart problems – *hart prob-lums* – medical conditions connected with the heart and the pumping and flow of *blood* around the body. They are a *contraindication* to some scalp massage techniques, such as *high frequency* treatments.

Heat damage – *heet dam-ij* – physical damage caused by heated *equipment*. The overuse of *straighteners*, *curling tongs* and *hairdryers* can adversely affect the *cuticle* of the hair.

Heat regulation – *heet reg-yoo-lay-shun* – the maintenance of body *temperature* at 37 degrees Celsius (98.6 degrees Fahrenheit) to allow the functions of the body to perform normally.

Heat testing materials – *heet tes-ting mu-teer-ee-ulz* – items used for testing the *temperature* of non-electrical equipment. For example, to check the heat level of a *pressing comb* when *thermally styling* the hair, the comb is placed on a tissue. If the tissue becomes scorched or burnt the comb is too hot and needs to be cooled before using it on the hair.

Heated rollers – *hee-td rol-urz* – electrical, heated styling *equipment* of various sizes which curl and add lift and *volume* to the hair. Made of plastic, each has an open middle and sits on a metal rod within a box that heats up the rollers. Hair is wound around each roller and allowed to cool, producing a soft *curl* in the hair.

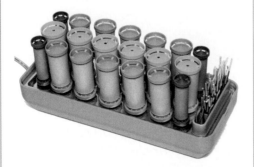

Heated rollers

High frequency – *hiy free-kw-ensee* – a type of scalp massage *service* using a piece of electrical *equipment*, which has an oscillating (moving back and forth), alternating current (flow), used to stimulate blood flow, improve the condition of the scalp and promote healthy hair growth. The unit can be used directly or indirectly on the scalp. Direct application uses a glass bulb over the scalp to conduct the current which increases cellular activity and dries up *seborrhoea* (oily scalp) or *dandruff*. Indirect application involves the client holding a glass rod (saturator) and the *stylist* conducting the current, whilst massaging the scalp. This method is warming and relaxing and soothes *nerve endings*. This specialist therapy makes a noise because of the changing current direction, so the client needs to be made aware of this prior to treatment.

High lift tint – *hiy lift tint* – a cream based *product* that lightens the hair up to 4–5 shades or levels of lightening. It is usually mixed one part tint to two parts *hydrogen peroxide* (although it is advisable to check the *manufacturer's instructions*). It is recommended for use on hair of a base 6 (dark blonde and above – see *depth*) and upwards. This type of product will not wash out of the hair so the colour will have to be grown out over a period of time.

High risk – *hiy risk* – of serious consequence or having great potential for harm.

Highlighting – *hiy-liyt-ing* – the process of **colouring** hair a lighter colour than the natural hair colour. Different methods can be used to lift the hair colour, for example, by using a *highlighting cap*, *spatula*, *foils* or *mesh*.

History of previous allergic reaction – *his-tu-ree ov pree-vee-us ul-ur-jik ree-ak-shun* – evidence of known *allergies* from the past. It is important to determine whether a client has reacted adversely to previous hairdressing treatments. For example, if a client has had a reaction to the glue used to bond *hair extensions*, it is highly probable that if the same glue is used again the client will have a similar reaction.

Hone – *h-own* – a tool used to sharpen *razors*. It is usually made of an abrasive (rough) material, which can be either natural, synthetic (man-made) or a combination of both. Natural ones are made from naturally occurring rock formations and require lubrication with continued...

Highlighting cap – *hiy-liyt-ing kap* – a strong flexible piece of plastic pierced with holes that is placed on the head when *highlighting* hair. Hair is pulled through the holes using a hook (available in various sizes) and then coloured, leaving the natural hair untouched underneath the cap.

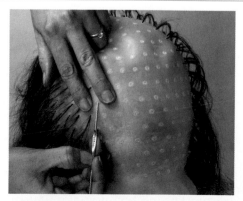

Highlighting cap

water or a *lathering product* before use. Synthetic ones can be used either wet or dry. Combination hones are a mixture of the two materials.

Hood dryer – *hud driy-ur* – electrically heated equipment that is used for drying hair. The client sits under a large dome from which hot air flows. This is regulated by a temperature control.

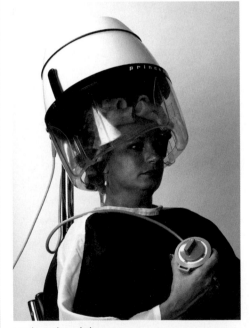

Under a hood dryer

Hopscotch perm winding – *hop-sk-och purm wiyn-ding* – a *perm winding* technique in which

perm rods are wound in the hair in different directions. This reduces the number of hair *partings* and creates *curls* going in various directions.

Hormone – *hor-mown* – a chemical released by *glands* in the body which causes cells to alter their activity. See also *acne vulgaris*.

Horny layer – *horn-ee lay-ur* – the top layer of the *epidermis* in the skin. This is the part of the skin which is visible on the body. The cells in this layer are flat, flaky and ready to be shed. They are composed mainly of *keratin* and overlap to protect the skin from damage. This layer of skin is thinnest on the eyelids and thickest on the feet. (See the structure of the skin diagram on page 159.)

Hot brush – *hot br-ush* – a piece of electrically heated *styling*

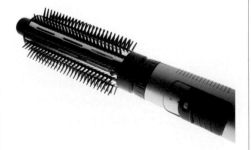

A hot brush

equipment, available in different sizes, used to produce different *curl* effects in the hair. It also adds lift and body to the hair.

Hot oil treatment – *hot oyl treet-mnt* – a treatment using a good quality oil with moisturising qualities, such as olive oil, which is applied to a dry scalp to nourish and add moisture to it. After the oil is warmed, it is applied and massaged into the scalp. An initial application of neat *shampoo* is massaged into the hair to emulsify the oil (distribute the oil particles) before adding water. Once all the oil is removed, the hair is shampooed and conditioned as normal.

Hot spots – *hot spo-tz* – areas on the head, such as the top of the head and the *nape*, that are naturally warmer than others. A *colouring* product or *perming* treatment will process more quickly in these parts.

Hot towel – *hot t-owl* – a towel that is warmed with moist heat and applied to the hair to soften the *cuticle* or to remove dirt and relax the client's face and muscles. It is usually placed in an electrical *steamer* unit to heat. Alternatively, it can be placed under hot running water and then wrung out to remove excess moisture. When applying a hot towel to the client's face it is important not to cover the nose to allow the client to breathe.

Human hair – *hyoo-mun hayr* – the natural hair that grows in *hair follicles* in the skin of humans. The hair on the head is sometimes cut and sold to be used as *hair extensions*.

Humidity – *hyoo-mid-it-ee* – moisture that is held within an atmosphere, such as in a damp environment or in the form of steam from hot baths. It changes the internal structure of the *hydrogen bonds* in hair from *beta keratin* (hair in its changed/stretched state) to *alpha keratin* (hair in its natural, un-stretched state).

Hydrogen bonds – *hiy-dro-jen bon-dz* – weak bonds found in the *molecular structure* of the *cortex* of the hair. Because they are temporary linkages the bonds can be broken down once the hair has been shampooed. This allows the hair to be stretched around a *roller* or brush. Once the hair has been stretched, fully dried and allowed to cool, the bonds become temporarily fixed *continued...*

into their new shape, changing straight hair into curly hair and curly hair into straight hair.

Hydrogen peroxide (H$_2$O$_2$) – *hiy-dro-jen pur-ox-iyd* – a *bleaching* and oxidising ingredient (see *oxidation*), found in hair bleach and *perm lotion*, and used to activate *quasi-permanent colour*, *permanent colour*, *highlighting* and bleaching products. Made from barium peroxide and diluted phosphoric acid, it is an unstable compound which is broken down into water and oxygen. It is available in various strengths and can be diluted using distilled water to achieve a particular strength. Its purpose is to soften and swell the *cuticle* to allow better *penetration* of the colour product. It causes oxygen to be released which activates the colour molecules. A 3% solution is used as an antiseptic and germicide (substances which destroy harmful *micro-organisms*) in mouthwash, but in full strength it can cause burns to the skin and mucous *membranes*. See also *Control of Substances Hazardous to Health Regulations 2002*.

Hygroscopic – *hiy-gro-skop-ik* – the ability to absorb water. When water is absorbed into the *cortex* the water breaks down the *hydrogen bonds*. This process allows the hair to be stretched. See also *beta keratin* and *alpha keratin*.

Hypersensitivity test – *hiy-pur-sens-i-tiv-it-ee test* – see *skin test*.

Identify – *iy-dent-if-iy* – to recognise or discover.

Identifying client needs – *iy-dent-if-iy-ing kliy-unt needz* – finding out about the requirements and expectations of a client. Hair type and suitability for a service can be established through asking the client *questions*, *visual check* of the scalp and hair, and performing tests on the hair. It also refers to pinpointing how to improve a salon's client services. See also *client needs*, *client requirements*, *client expectations*.

Illustrate – *il-us-tray-t* – to *explain* something by giving examples.

Image – *im-ij* – a representation of something, for example, a look from the punk rock or 1960s era.

Immunisation – *im-yoo-ni-zay-shun* – the process of making an individual immune or resistant to *disease*. It combats the most common diseases such as measles, rubella, mumps, *diphtheria*, polio and *whooping cough*. By injecting a vaccine (a solution containing a very small amount of the disease) into the *blood* stream it stimulates the body to produce its own antibodies against the disease. Exposure to the actual disease can also build up immunity, which protects in later life: a child suffering chickenpox will be uncomfortable whilst in the *pustule* stages, but then is protected against getting a more dangerous form of the disease (shingles) in later life.

Impetigo – *im-pe-tiy-go* – a common skin *disease* caused by a bacterial *infection*, seen as *pustules* which become crusted, usually around the mouth and nostrils. It can also occur on the scalp. It is highly *contagious* and a *medical referral* should be given. (See infectious diseases of the skin and scalp on pages 162–163.)

Implement – *im-plu-ment* – to bring about, for example, carrying out the implementation of a new *cutting* technique learnt at a training event.

Implementing instructions – *im-plu-ment-ing in-str-uk-shunz* – carrying out actions based upon a set of *instructions*, sometimes given or taught by someone.

Implication – *im-pli-kay-shun* – an indication of something that may not be immediately obvious or is not stated.

Incompatible – *in-kom-pat-u-bul* – not suitable.

Incompatibility test – *in-kom-pat-u-bil-it-ee test* – a test carried out before **colouring** and **perming** to show whether there are chemicals present in the hair that contain **metallic salts**. Metallic salts will react with the **hydrogen peroxide** in the salon colour treatment, which may cause the hair to fall apart and/or cause scalp burns. To test hair, a solution of hydrogen peroxide and alkaline **perm lotion** is mixed and a small cutting of hair is placed in the solution. After thirty minutes if there is no change in the hair and no reaction in the bowl it is safe to carry out the colour treatment. If the liquid

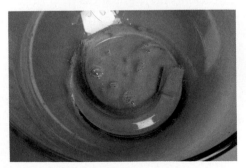

The incompatibility test

fizzes and the hair colour changes or the bowl generates a lot of heat, there are chemicals already in the hair which make it unsuitable for further treatment.

Incompatible product – *in-kom-pat-u-bul pro-duk-t* – a **product** that does not work with other products. It may cause a reaction that could damage the hair and skin. See also *incompatibility test*.

Incorporate – *in-kor-por-ayt* – to take in or include as part of a whole. An example is to add hair **ornamentation** to **enhance** a hairstyle for a wedding or ball.

Incorrect completion – *in-kor-ekt kom-plee-shun* – a term usually applied to a **cheque** which has not been filled out correctly. The cheque is returned from the bank stating it cannot be drawn against, because some detail is missing.

Increase salon business – *in-k-rees sa-lon biz-nis* – produce a higher than usual turnover of clients and income by generating new and repeat business, and through an increase in sales of retail **products**. See also **takings**.

Infection – *in-fek-shun* – the successful invasion, establishment and growth of *micro-organisms* to a degree that causes symptoms of a disease. It can be caused by *bacteria*, *viruses* or *fungi* which are too small to be seen with the naked eye but are always present in the environment. (*Parasites* also cause infection.) Hairdressers are mostly concerned with recognising infectious *contagious* diseases, so as not to spread them from one client to another or to themselves. The discovery of some diseases will be a *contraindication* to treatment. A *medical referral* should be recommended. (See infectious diseases of the skin and scalp on pages 162–163.)

Infestation – *in-fest-ay-shun* – a term applied to *parasites* which live in or on another living creature in large numbers. The most common one found in hairdressing is *head lice*.

Infill colour – *in-fil kul-ur* – a colour that is placed in-between *foils*, *mesh* or *wraps*, usually following the same method as a *full head application*. It is often used if a client has a high percentage of *white hair* but still likes a combination of colours.

Inflammation – *in-flam-ay-shun* – a *condition* in which the affected part of the body becomes swollen, hot and sometimes painful. See also *acne*.

Inform – *in-form* – to notify, such as telling a manager about any complaints that a client has made, or informing clients about any changes to the services offered.

Information – *in-form-ay-shun* – knowledge gained by speaking with someone, by studying and/or through experience. A client in a salon will need to know about timings and outcomes of *services*, and prices of services and *products*. However, it is important that the hairdresser is aware of the legal *implications* of information given out. See also *Trade Descriptions Act 1968 and 1972*.

In-growing hair – *in-grow-ing hayr* – any hair which has grown back in on itself and has burrowed underneath the skin's surface. It is usually short and curly, and is commonly found along the *nape*, due to friction (rubbing) of a shirt collar on the skin, and in the beard continued...

area, through **shaving**. It is not painful unless **infection** sets in and **pus** forms in the area. If this is the case a **medical referral** to a **General Practitioner** should be recommended. Regular **exfoliation** of the skin and massage prevents this condition to some degree.

In-house – in-how-s – within a **workplace**, company or organisation.

Injury – in-jur-ee – evidence of damage to a person. If the skin on the scalp is broken, bruised or damaged, this is a **contraindication** to some scalp massage techniques, such as **high frequency** services.

Innovative – in-no-vu-tiv – new methods or ideas, for example, changing the way **tools** and **equipment** are used to achieve different results.

Inspect – in-spek-t – to examine. For example, it is important to inspect the details of a credit card, especially if there may be a suspicion that something is not correct.

Insurance – in-shoor-uns – a system of providing financial protection against specific unforeseen events, such as fire, death, loss or damage. A specialist insurance company provides a policy in return for a premium (regular payment) for such protection. Nearly all areas of hairdressing can be insured: loss of earnings should an employee become ill, theft of tools and equipment, fire, flooding and so on. The more insurance cover that is required, the higher the premium payments will be.

All hairdressers should at least have:

1. Professional Indemnity Insurance – this is for protection against any claim made by a client for injury or damage caused by a treatment. Employees should not assume that their employer has this insurance cover, so it is wise to provide their own cover to protect against any claims personally made against them.

2. Public Liability Insurance – this will protect the salon owner should anything happen to a client whilst on the business premises. This is not compulsory, but certainly

advisable to protect against any compensation claim.

Instruction – *in-str-uk-shun* – the giving of directions through teaching or training. Being attentive when instruction is given ensures correct development of techniques and the learning of new skills to avoid harming the client – especially when dealing with chemical processes.

Intensive massage – *in-ten-siv mas-arj* – deep, stimulating massage using *petrissage* massage movements.

Internal Verification – *in-tur-nul veri-fi-kay-shun* – a college's internal system which ensures that its process of assessment is fair and uniform across all groups and all assessors. The role of an *Internal Verifier* (IV) is to cross-check all groups' assessment portfolios and ensure that the right type and amount of evidence is put forward to an *External Verification* body.

Internal Verifier – *in-tur-nul veri-f-iy-ur* – a person (often called an IV) appointed by a college to manage the assessment process to ensure that key skills

are being assessed at the same national standard. See also *Internal Verification*.

International colour chart (ICC) – *intur-na-shun-ul kul-ur ch-art* – a shade (colour) chart showing all the colours in the ranges for specific colouring manufacturers. Although each manufacturer has a slightly different system, all companies number the basic hair colours from 1–10: 1 being the darkest (black) and 10 being the lightest (lightest blonde). See also *depth*.

Intertwine – *in-tur-twiyn* – to twist together, such as when twisting *yarn locks* into existing hair. See also *plaiting*.

Invalid card – *in-val-id kard* – a debit or credit card from which payment is unable to be made, or is refused *authorisation*. The reasons for this may be that the card is out of date, the client has inputted the wrong PIN number, or the client's signature does not match the signature on the card. See also *counterfeit*.

Invalid currency – *in-val-id kur-en-see* – a form of payment which is not recognised as *legal tender*. See also *cash*.

73

Job responsibilities – *job rus-pon-su-bil-it-eez* – specific duties related to a job. For example, as well as hairdressing duties, a person, if specially trained in safe evacuation duties, may be the fire officer for the salon.

Job role – *Jub rol* – a person's duties as outlined within a *contract of employment*. For *health and safety* reasons, it is important that people in a salon do not exceed the powers of their authority.

Keloids – *kee-loydz* – an overgrowth of **scar tissue** found on the skin. It is a firm, shiny mass of fibrous tissue, often raised, which forms at the site of a burn, wound or surgical incision. It is most commonly found on skins with high **pigmentation**, such as African Caribbean skin. If it causes discomfort, or there is deterioration in the **condition**, further growth, or it changes shape, a **medical referral** to a **General Practitioner** or a **dermatologist** is advised before the problem worsens. Although this is a non-infectious condition, there is risk of **infection** if the skin is damaged. See also **melanin**.

Keratin – *ker-a-tin* – an insoluble protein found in horny tissue in the outer layer of skin (see **horny layer**), the hair and the nails. It is found in the **cuticle** cells of hair and it makes the hair elastic and flexible. In the skin and nails it toughens the cells and makes them waterproof. Non-keratinised cells are found in moist areas of the body, such as the mouth.

Keratinisation – *ker-a-tin-iy-zay-shun* – the formation of **keratin** in body tissue.

Knot – *n-ot* – a fastening made by passing the ends of a section of hair through a loop and pulling them tight. It is a dressing technique used for **styling** medium to longer length hair. A number of different effects can be produced when knots are tied with pieces of cloth, string or ribbon. For example, a big knot made with a large section of hair will create a casual, loose effect.

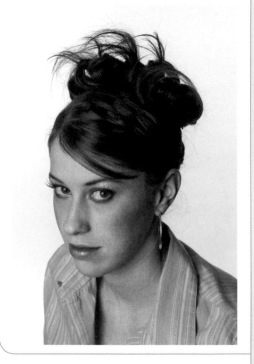

Knowledge – *no-lij* – information or facts. In relation to hairdressing, it is recalling appropriate, previously continued...

learned information and applying it in a practical way, such as using skills when carrying out *services*, discussing *products* with the client and assessing *client needs*.

Knowledge evidence – *no-lij ev-i-duns* – proof of *knowledge* that underpins a particular task and explains *what*, *when*, *where*, *why*, *who*, *how* and *what if*. This can be shown in the performance of a task, through answering *questions* in distance learning packs, through projects or on written papers. See also *assessment*.

Lanugo hair – *lan-oo-go hayr* – see *hair types*.

Lathering product – *lar-thur-ing pro-duk-t* – any soap-based product, in the form of foam, *gel* or solid blocks of soap, used during a *shaving service*. When wet, it produces a soft foamy substance which is used to lubricate, remove dirt from, and soften the skin.

Layering – *lay-ur-ing* – *cutting* the inner lengths of hair (not the perimeter edge of the hair) to produce shape and movement in a haircut.

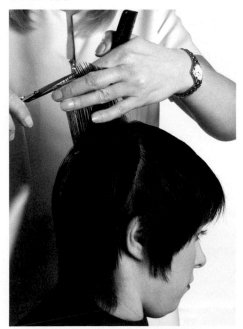

Layering

Legal duty – *lee-gul dyoo-tee* – a duty which must be carried out by law. It is laid down under *legislation* mainly to protect people within a *workplace*.

Legal requirement – *lee-gul re-kw-iyr-mnt* – a rule as laid down by *legislation*. If a person (or a company) does not abide by this, he or she is liable to prosecution which can result in fines, imprisonment and/or hefty compensation claims from employees and clients. In a business, there are many, which regulate the way the business is operated, how the *workplace* is set up and managed, how people are employed and what systems of working must be used. See also *legislation*.

Legal tender – *lee-gul ten-dur* – *cash* in the form of coins and banknotes which are acceptable as a form of payment by law within a country.

Legislation – *lej-is-lay-shun* – laws that have been made for the protection of all in society and business. (See legislation on pages 164–165.)

Length – *len-g-th* – the measurement or extent of

something from one end to the other. For example, if the hair sits above the shoulders, it is considered short; if it is below the shoulders, it is classed as long.

Lightening product – *liy-tun-ing pro-duk-t* – any **product** that has the ability to lighten the hair's natural colour, such as a **permanent colour**, **high lift tint** or **bleach**.

Limitations of treatment – *lim-it-ay-shunz ov treet-mnt* – the restrictions which apply to a treatment. It is important to understand and describe what a treatment will do for the client. For example, a haircut resembling a celebrity's hairstyle will not make the client look like the celebrity, but it may add shape and definition to the client's hair. See also **client needs** and **client expectations**.

Limits of own authority – *lim-itz ov own or-th-or-it-ee* – the limits to which a person can make decisions or give orders. This may be laid down in the job description or be part of the **policies** in the **workplace** which state what someone can and cannot do in relation to a job or duty.

Line manager – *liy-n man-uj-ur* – a senior member who is responsible for managing a particular employee. For example, a person in a salon management team who is responsible for giving an **employee** appraisals.

Link selling – *link sel-ing* – **selling** related items. For example, recommending to the client products which **complement** each other, such as a particular **conditioner** which goes with a **shampoo**.

Listening skills – *lis-un-ing sk-ilz* – ability to pay attention through listening. Effective listening includes showing interest in the person talking, responding in an appropriate manner, nodding one's head, maintaining eye contact and sharing empathy with the talker.

Local bylaws – *lo-kul biy-lorz* – laws set by the local authority. As they may vary from other local authorities, it is important to establish which area a salon or venue comes under so that **employees** are familiar with any **legal duties**.

Lock – *lok* – a single section of hair which is manipulated or twisted and left to form or grow.

Locking – *lok-ing* – (also known as 'locksing') *twisting* the client's natural hair using a single twisting method. It is advisable to get the client to visit the salon as the hair grows to separate the *locks* and continue the twisting process in the root area. The smaller the section taken, the tighter the twist. It is important not to over twist or twist the hair too tightly as this may result in hair loss. Having long, heavy locks can also lead to hair loss. See also *dreadlocks*.

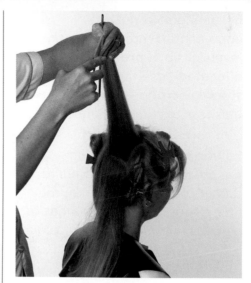

Removing length at the crown

Locking stages for cultivating lock:

Budding Stage: Hair begins to interlace and mesh to form the first stage of the locking process.

Growing Stage: Hair strands interlace to form a firm unit.

Mature Stage: The lock is now totally entwined to give a tighter rope-like look.

Long graduation – *long grad-yoo-ay-shun* – when the inner layers of the hair *lengths* are shorter than the outline shape (perimeter edge) of a haircut. See also *short graduation*.

Loss of depth – *los ov dep-th* – when the original *base colour* becomes lighter than the original *target colour*.

Lotion – *lo-shun* – a liquid preparation. It protects the hair from *atmospheric moisture* by coating it with a plastic resin that acts as a barrier. Spirit-based *blow-drying* lotions or medium-to-firm hold *setting* lotions are sprayed or sprinkled from a bottle on to wet hair prior to a drying service.

Low level – *lo lev-ul* – a low or minimum amount. In a salon, to prevent items *continued...*

becoming sold out, it is important to maintain *stock* levels of each *product* above its allocated base number. Regular *stock control* is essential for the business to function smoothly.

Lowlighting – *lo-liyt-ing* – the process of *colouring* hair a darker colour than the natural hair colour. Different methods can be used to darken the hair colour, for example, by using a cap, *spatula*, *foils* or *mesh*.

Low risk – *lo risk* – of minimal consequence, or having little or no potential for harm. However, caution should always be taken in any situation.

Lye – *liy* – an *alkaline* solution which is sodium-based having a *pH* of between 9 and 14. It is found in *sodium relaxers*.

Machinery – *mush-een-ur-ree* – mechanical or electrical devices which help to perform tasks. Examples within the hairdressing trade are **steamers**, **climazones** and **high frequency** units.

Maintenance – *mayn-ten-uns* – the continuation of something at the same level. Keeping up a hairstyle, for example, depends on how much time, money and ability a client has to do this. Some styles will need the use of **styling** products and heated electrical **equipment** (e.g. **straighteners**) to ensure it looks how it should and your client needs to be able to maintain the look every day. Some hairdressing **services** will need to be performed regularly, such as a re-application of **colouring** products, or regular **cutting**, in order to keep the hair looking good.

Make-up – *may-kup* – cosmetic **products** used on the face, for example, eye shadow, mascara, lipstick, to improve its appearance. The cosmetics chosen need to **complement** the overall image being created. See also **make-up artist**.

Make-up artist – *may-kup art-ist* – a person trained in the art

of applying **make-up** to create different looks. The artist works at hairdressing photo shoots and to **enhance** the overall image created during a **hair show** or **competition work**.

Male pattern baldness – *mayl pat-urn borl-d-nes* – see **androgenic alopecia**.

Manage – *man-ij* – to deal or cope with, or to control something; to give direction or advice to someone.

Manager – *man-uj-ur* – a person who oversees or takes charge of a situation, for example, the staff and **resources** in a salon.

Mandatory units – *man-dut-or-ee yoo-nits* – **units** within a study course which are compulsory and must be achieved to gain a **qualification**.

Manual Handling Operations Regulations 1992 – *man-yoo-ul hand-ling op-ur-ay-shunz reg-yoo-lay-shunz* – this **legislation** is to do with the handling or lifting of heavy loads, which may include equipment or boxes of stock. A **risk assessment** should *continued...*

be undertaken and safe systems of work put into place, for all to follow.

Manufacturer's instructions – *man-yoo-fak-tyu-rurs in-struk-shunz* – important details supplied by the company of a product to explain how to use a product correctly. They should always be read and followed for *health and safety* reasons. Misusing or ignoring these may give grounds for a *negligence* charge, should it be proven that an *employee* endangered a client's health and safety through incorrect use. See also *Provision and Use of Work Equipment Regulations 1998*.

Marketing – *mar-kut-ing* – advertising, promoting or *selling* something, for example, a salon advertising to a target audience where there may be a demand for particular *services*, such as *plaiting* or *braiding*, in an African Caribbean community.

Massage – *mas-arj* – to manipulate (move, treat) the skin in order to relax *nerve endings* and stimulate *sebaceous glands* and *blood supply*, thereby increasing oxygen and nutrients to feed the hair.

Massage media – *mas-arj mee-dee-ur* – *products* applied to the scalp to aid massage services.

Materials – *mat-eyr-ee-ulz* – *equipment* needed to carry out a task, for example, a comb, *scissors* and *clippers* for a *beard trim*.

Matrix – *may-tri-x* – see *germinal matrix*.

Measuring flask – *me-zhr-ing flar-sk* – a clear cylinder marked with measurements in millilitres used to measure out products, for example, *hydrogen peroxide* for a *colouring* service.

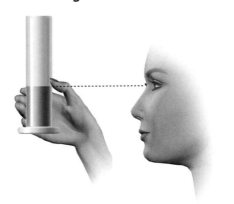

Accurately reading the amount in a measuring flask

Mechanical handling device – *mek-an-i-kul hand-ling du-viys* –

an aid for lifting heavy *equipment*, such as a forklift truck used in a warehouse. Untrained persons must not use this before proper training is given and a *risk assessment* is carried out.

Medical advice – *med-ik-ul ad-viys* – advice relating to a client's medical condition. Factors such as the prescribed drugs a client is taking, or a medical treatment the client is having, need to be taken into account when carrying out a hairdressing *service*, especially one involving the use of chemicals. See also *contra-indication* and *chemotherapy*.

Medulla – *med-ul-ur* – the central part of the *hair shaft*. It is made up of soft cells with air spaces in-between them but is not known to have any particular function. It can be missing in very fine hair. (See the hair follicle diagram on page 159.)

Medical referral – *med-ik-ul ru-fur-ul* – directing someone to a specialist to investigate a particular medical problem. It is important that a hairdresser can recognise various *skin disorders* and *diseases*, and the differences between those that do not need specialist treatment and those that require the client to consult a *trichologist*, *General Practitioner*, *dermatologist* or a *pharmacist*. Hairdressers should not name specific conditions as they have not had medical training and may cause unnecessary stress to the client. (See infectious diseases of the skin and scalp on pages 162–163.)

Melanin – *mel-u-nin* – the hair's natural colour *pigment* found in the *cortex*. It is broken down into two types of pigments: *eumelanin* – black/brown, and *pheomelanin* – yellow and red. It varies in quantity and accounts for the racial differences in skin and hair colour. The lighter someone's hair, the less melanin there is. In the skin it is found in cells called melanocytes, contained in the *basal layer* of the *epidermis*.

Membrane – *mem-br-ayn* – a thin, soft, pliable sheet of tissue that lines a tube or cavity, covering organs and structures of the body. There are four types within the body:

1. serous (lines cavities and forming outer layers of organs)
2. mucous (lines tubes, such as those of the digestive system)

continued…

3. cutaneous (the *epidermis* of the skin)
4. synovial (lines joints to allow movement).

Mesh – *me-sh* – a clear plastic, re-useable packet of various sizes used for *colouring* hair. It has an adhesive strip at the top to allow the packet to stick together when closed. It is usually used for *weaving* techniques rather than for *slicing* of colour because it is difficult for the adhesive to hold together if used with a solid block of hair. It is transparent to allow the *stylist* to monitor the development of the colour more easily.

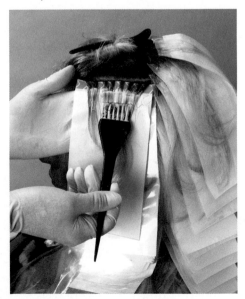

Using meshes during colouring

Mesh of hair – *me-sh ov hayr* – 1. a section of hair that is taken to suit the size of a *roller* or *perm rod*. 2. a section of hair used for *weaving* colour through hair.

Metallic salts – *me-ta-lik sol-tz* – tiny pieces of metal within some home *colouring products*. These are not *compatible* with professional colouring products and may cause hair damage.

Method of payment – *meth-ud ov pay-mnt* – a way of making a payment. In a salon, a client can choose to pay for the service provided using *cash*, a *cheque*, a *credit card* or a *debit card*, or gift *vouchers*.

Micro-organisms – *miy-kro-or-gun-iz-mz* – organisms that are too small to be seen with the naked eye, such as *bacteria*, *fungi* and *viruses*. Microbes are single-celled organisms which cause *disease*.

Mitosis – *miy-to-sis* – the process whereby cells divide and make exact copies of themselves. In relation to hair growth, it occurs within the *dermal papilla* of the skin. Uneven cell division is thought to contribute towards curly hair formation, as one side of the **hair shaft** develops faster than the other.

Modification – *mod-i-fi-kay-shun* – the adaptation of a service to take into account varying, and sometimes unexpected, factors. For example, a cut or abrasion on the scalp may mean that an 'off scalp' *colouring* application will need to be done using a **highlighting cap**, **foils** or **mesh**.

Moisturiser – *moy-s-chur-iy-zur* – a product that adds moisture to the hair. Serums and other oil-based products will reduce dryness, **frizziness** and give shine to the hair.

Molecular structure – *mol-ek-yoo-lur struk-chur* – the **molecules** that make up the structure of something. Hair is made up of a protein called **keratin**. Chemically, it is a series of amino acids and peptides, which, when joined together, make polypeptide chains. These are further supported by **hydrogen bonds** (which are easily broken by water) and **disulphide bonds** (which can only be broken by other chemicals).

Molecule – *mol-u-kyool* – a chemical combination of a group of **atoms** bonded together.

Moulding (stage) – *mol-ding* – one of the three stages of **perming** hair. After the **perm lotion** opens and swells the **cuticle** (softening stage), it enters the **cortex** where it deposits hydrogen. The hydrogen attaches itself to the **disulphide bonds** and breaks them apart into sulphur bonds. (Not all disulphide bonds are broken during perming.) The hair is now able to take on the shape of the perm rod.

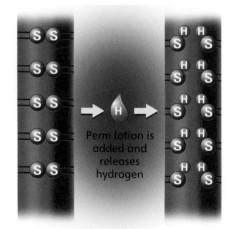
Perm lotion is added and releases hydrogen

The moulding stage

Mousse – *moo-s* – a **product**, used for **styling** hair, available in pumps or pressurised continued...

85

cans, which foams up after making contact with air. It gives a light-to-firm or extra-firm hold, and is used to give body and bounce to the hair. Applied to wet hair, it protects the hair from *atmospheric moisture*.

Moustache trim – *mus-t-a-sh trim* – the **cutting** of facial hair above the top lip. The hair is combed into place and the required *length* over the lip is cut using *scissors* and the *freehand* method. Once evenness of hair length is checked, the *scissor-over-comb* or *clipper-over-comb* technique can be used to remove bulk and length from the remaining moustache hair. It is important not to remove the hair that is shaped to extend past the area of actual growth.

Nape – *nay-p* – the back of the neck.

Nape whorl – *nay-p wurl* – a particular *hair growth pattern* at the *nape* of the neck, in which the hair grows in circles rather than straight across. As the hairline is uneven, care must be taken not to cut above it.

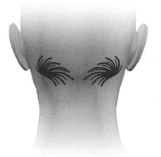

Nape whorls hair growth pattern

National Occupational Standards (NOS) – *nash-nul ok-yoo-pay-shun-ul stan-durds* – statements of performance, recognised nationally, which cover the skills, knowledge and understanding needed to undertake a particular job. The correct level of tasks and competencies are set as *units* and are used to design *National Vocational Qualifications* (NVQs). These are set by the lead bodies in consultation with hairdressing companies and salon owners to determine which skills are required within the commercial industry.

National Vocational Qualification (NVQ) – *nash-nul vo-kay-shun-ul kwal-i-fi-kay-shun* – work-related, competence-based qualification, which reflects the skills needed to do a job effectively, allowing candidates to prove they are competent for employment. Each *qualification* is a collection of completed *units*, giving sufficient evidence to cover all requirements within an assessment book. The units are completed over a period of time and are carried out only in recognised salons, or colleges with the correct *Awarding Body* approval and verification system.

Natural parting – *nat-yoor-ul par-ting* – the way in which hair falls naturally. It can produce a middle, off-centre or side *parting*.

Natural pigmentation – *nat-yoor-ul pig-men-tay-shun* – the hair's natural colour made up of a combination of any of the four main hair colour pigments known as *melanin* (red, yellow, black and brown).

Necessary tests – *nes-us-ury tests* – tests which are essential to carry out. In hairdressing, *observation* is made of test results to *assess* the hair and scalp, and give proper *treatment* advice to the client. Examples include a *porosity test* (or *texture test*), an *elasticity test*, an *incompatibility test*, a *skin test* and *test cutting*. It is important to use salon guidelines and procedures when carrying out pre-service testing and to follow the *manufacturer's instructions*.

Neck brush – *nek br-ush* – a brush used throughout a *haircut* to remove unwanted hair cuttings from the face, ears and neck.

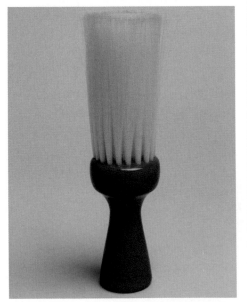

A neck brush

Neckline shape – *nek-liyn shay-p* – the shape of the hairline created around the neck area. It is determined by the client's natural hairline and the look they want to achieve. There is no specific neckline shape for each *haircut*. See *rounded neckline*, *square neckline*, *tapered neckline*.

Negative – *neg-a-tiv* – not *positive*, uncooperative. In a salon it is important not to give poor responses or display body language which reflects an uninterested attitude towards clients and colleagues. If so, it may be necessary for the salon management members to plan and *implement* changes to improve *customer services*.

Negative reaction – *neg-a-tiv ree-ak-shun* – no positive reaction. When a client has no reaction to hair and skin tests performed before a *perm* or *colouring* service, the *service* can continue to be carried out.

Negligence – *neg-li-jens* – failure to attend properly to duties.

Negotiate – *ne-go-sh-ee-ayt* – to consult with someone and reach an agreement on something.

Nerve endings – *nurv end-ingz* – receptors in the skin. They send messages to and from the brain so that the body can react appropriately to stimulus outside the body. For example, when touching something hot, a person will pull away from the heat for protection. Sensations that are felt by the skin are touch, pain, heat and cold, pressure and itchiness. See also **hair nerves**. (See the structure of the skin diagram on page 159.)

Neutralise – *nyoo-tra-liyz* – to make neutral or ineffective.

Neutralise colour tone – *nyoo-tra-liyz kul-ur tow-n* – to *neutralise* an unwanted hair tone. For example, if the hair contains too much warmth, the opposite colour on the colour wheel would be chosen to counterbalance this. See also **colour wheel**.

Neutraliser – *nyoo-tra-liyz-ur* – chemical used to *neutralise* hair.

Neutralising – *nyoo-tra-liyz-ing* – the chemical process used to fix hair in a new position (permanently) after it has been altered by the action of **perm lotion**. The chemicals remove

hydrogen from the **cortex** by adding oxygen (a process of **oxidation**). This process joins together the sulphur bonds to re-form **disulphide bonds** in a new position, permanently fixing the curl.

Neutralising shampoo – *nyoo-tra-liyz-ing sham-poo* – a **shampoo** used after chemically **relaxing** the hair to fix the hair permanently in its new position. After the **relaxing product** has processed, the hair is rinsed and the shampoo is added. The shampoo restores the hair's natural **pH** balance, closes the **cuticle** and helps remove any remaining relaxer.

Nine section perm winding – *niyn sek-shun purm wiyn-ding* – a traditional technique which involves dividing the hair neatly into **nine sections** and winding **perm rods** into them. Usually winding starts from the central secton of the **nape** area, and then continues in the left and right nape sections. The central and left and right crown sections are then wound, followed lastly by the central top section, and both left and right side sections. This allows a good fit to the head avoiding **root drag**.

Nine sections – *niyn sek-shunz* – a term used for the division of hair into nine sections in preparation for **perm winding**. See also **nine section perm winding**.

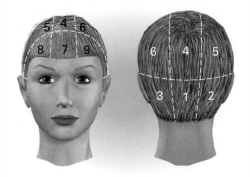

Nine sections of the head

Non-cash payment – *non-kash pay-mnt* – a payment made using gift **vouchers**, a **credit card** or a **debit card**, or a **cheque**.

Non-conventional items – *non-kon-ven-shun-ul i-tums* – non-traditional items, for example, hair **accessories** such as chopsticks, or pieces of fabric, that are not usually used for **ornamentation** in long hair-up styles.

Non-sodium relaxer – *non-so-dee-um ru-lax-ur* – a **relaxing product** classified as a no-**lye** product which is less irritating to the scalp and **penetrates** the **cuticle** slowly. However, it causes

the hair to dry out and so the hair will need frequent conditioning treatments. See also **sodium relaxer**.

Normal (hair or scalp) – *nor-mul* – hair or scalp that is neither dry nor greasy and has a normal or even **porosity**.

NOS – *en-o-es* – short for **National Occupational Standards**.

Notched scissors – *not-ch-d siz-urz* – see **thinning scissors**.

Notifiable disease – *no-t-if-iy-a-bul diz-eez* – a **disease** which, by law, must be reported to a health authority. (See infectious diseases of the skin and scalp on pages 162–163.)

Nozzle – *noz-ul* – a plastic attachment, wide at one end that fits onto a **hairdryer** and narrow at the other to direct the **airflow** from the hairdryer to a certain part of the hair. Because the heat is directed to a specific area, it prevents the rest of the hair from being blown around and dries the hair more quickly.

NVQ – *en-vee-kyoo* – short for **National Vocational Qualification**.

Objective – *ob-j-ek-tiv* – a goal or aim to work towards. For example, an *S/NVQ* candidate's personal goal is to move forward to the next level of development, and a salon's target might be to attract more clients to increase revenue coming into the business. See also *SMART targets*.

Oblong face shape – *ob-long fay-s shay-p* – a narrow *head and face shape*. Width is needed to make the face appear shorter. A *fringe* would be suitable with short hair. Asymmetric (unbalanced) styles also suit this face shape. (See head and face shapes on page 161.)

Observe – *obs-er-v* – closely watch or monitor something or someone.

Observational skills – *obs-er-vay-shun-ul sk-ils* – the skills used to *observe* something or someone carefully. Examples include examining the hair and scalp, or studying a client's reaction or response during a *consultation*. See also *visual check*, *necessary tests*.

Oils – *oylz* – *finishing products* designed to add moisture and give maximum shine to the hair. Care must be taken not to use excess amounts of these products as they will make the hair greasy and lank. They are not suitable to use on hair that is naturally greasy.

One length – *wun leng-th* – hair that is cut to the same *length* around the outside or perimeter edge of the hair.

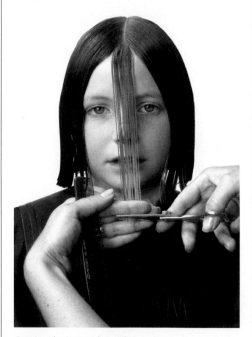

Cutting hair one length

Open blade razor – *o-pun bl-ay-d ray-zur* – see *cut-throat razor*.

Open questions – *o-pun kw-es-chun-z* – questions requiring full answers, rather than just a 'yes' or a 'no' answer. They help to keep the conversation flowing during a **consultation**. See also **questions** and **closed questions**.

Optional units – *op-shun-ul yoo-nits* – **units** which are not mandatory (compulsory), but add to a **qualification**. An **S/NVQ** candidate's college or **assessment** centre will have chosen the most suitable pathway to give maximum employment potential, guiding the candidate towards the units he or she needs to take. The front of an assessment book shows the mandatory and optional unit pathway.

Oral questions – *or-ul kwes-chunz* – spoken questions. An **assessor** may ask **S/NVQ** candidates questions to prove their level of understanding and to clarify points brought up during the **assessment** process. The evidence from these will be recorded and it may cover a range or performance criteria that were not covered during **direct observation**.

Ordering system – *or-d-ur-ing sis-tum* – the process of arranging for **stock** to be sent to a business from **product** suppliers. A salon usually holds stock sheets which list the code number, name, details and numbers left of each stock item. **Low levels** of items indicate that these are good selling lines and more are required. Ordering can take place in person, over the phone, by fax, email or letter. Some companies have representatives who visit salons and order the items with you. Most wholesale companies like the salon to have an account with them and to use the correct forms when filling in orders.

Organisation – *org-un-iy-zay-shun* – an establishment or an industry-related institute which provides **professional** membership.

Ornamentation – *orn-u-men-tay-shun* – any object used to add interest, beauty or detail. **Accessories** attached to hair are used to **complement** a style or look. For example, a ribbon can be threaded through a **plait** to give a greater impact; chopsticks can be inserted into a **French pleat** to add interest; beads can be used on the end of plaits to hide unruly ends and add colour to the hair.

Other persons – *u-thur pur-sunz* – a phrase referring to people, other than business employees, covered under the *Health and Safety at Work Act 1974* who enter the premises of work or training establishment/college such as clients and potential clients, contractors, sales persons, *product* suppliers, students, models, visitors and members of the public.

Outcome – *ow-t-kum* – the consequence of an action, such as the result of *product* sales, a salon's goal or a personal achievement.

Outline – *ow-t-liyn* – the outside edge defined by the shape of a *hairstyle*, beard, moustache or *sideburns*.

Oval face shape – *o-vul fay-s shay-p* – a *head and face shape* which is considered to have the ideal bone structure and shape for any hairstyle. The chin tapers gently from a slightly wider forehead. (See head and face shapes on page 161.)

Oven – *u-vun* – see *thermal heating stove*.

Over-dry – *o-vur-driy* – to use electrical tools excessively to remove excess moisture from the hair. As the moisture has been removed from the hair the *hydrogen bonds* will have re-formed, so it will not be possible to alter the physical shape. Over-use of heat effectively 'bakes' the hair and causes dryness and damage to the hair.

Overheads – *o-vur-hedz* – essential expenses incurred in the running of a business such as rent, rates, heating, laundry, all utilities, including telephone, electricity and gas, wages, and *equipment* purchase and *maintenance*. See also *resources*.

Over-processing – *o-vur-pro-ses-ing* – exceeding the development time of a *chemical service*. This can cause deterioration of the hair.

Overtrading – *o-vur-tray-ding* – a situation in which a business is trading more than it can afford to finance – in simple terms, when it has more money going out of it than it is bringing in. See also *profit*.

Oxidation – *ox-i-day-shun* – a chemical process that *continued...*

93

Oxidation

involves combining a substance with oxygen. It occurs in *permanent colour* and *quasi-permanent colour* processes, *bleaching* and when *neutralising* a perm. The oxygen used in these processes comes from *hydrogen peroxide*. The chemicals in the *neutraliser* remove the hydrogen from the *cortex* by adding oxygen.

Palm rolling – *p-arm ro-ling* – a method used for grooming *locks* to create a uniform look. It takes advantage of the hair's natural ability to coil.

Papule – *pap-yool* – a small, solid, round lump raised on the skin's surface, commonly referred to as a pimple.

Para dye – *pa-ra diy* – another term given to synthetic (man-made) *permanent colour*.

Parasite – *par-a-siyt* – an organism that lives in or on another organism and gets its nourishment from its host. An *infestation* caused by a parasitic invasion can cause *infection*, such as *head lice*.

Partial head – *par-shul hed* – a *service* which is carried out on part of the hair rather than the *full head*, for example, when a colour is applied to a specific section of hair to create an effect, or when some of the hair is plaited.

Parting – *part-ing* – a line or division in the hair created by combing sections away from it. There are different types: straight, long, short, zig-zag, diagonal, centre, side.

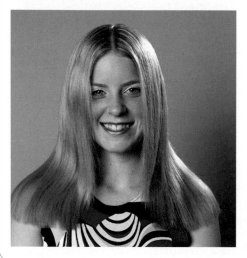

Patch test – *pach test* – see *skin test*.

Payment card – *pay-mnt kard* – see *credit card* and *debit card*.

Payment dispute – *pay-mnt dis-pyoo-t* – a problem or a disagreement over a payment. Examples include receiving *counterfeit* money or an invalid *credit card* or *debit card* from a client, or when a client has not filled out a *cheque* correctly.

Pear face shape – *p-ayr fay-s shay-p* – a *head and face shape* which is determined by a narrow forehead with the face gradually widening to the angle of the jaw which is broad and prominent. The ideal hairstyle for this shape should create the impression of width across the forehead and make the jaw line seem narrower. The hair should be swept off the forehead to create an illusion of width. (See head and face shapes on page 161.)

Penetrate – *pen-u-tray-t* – to enter or pass through.

to the original colour of the hair. It is important to determine whether the client has 0–10%, 10–20%, 20–30% and so on of this type of hair to help decide the right amount of *base colour* to add to ensure complete coverage of the white hair.

Performance Criteria (PC) – *pur-form-uns kriy-teyr-eeya* – statements explaining how particular activities or tasks should be done to show an *S/NVQ* candidate's competence. Boxes in the candidate's *assessment* book are ticked only when the

Penetrating conditioner – *pen-u-tray-ting kon-dish-un-ur* – a conditioning product that smoothes and coats *cuticle* scales and penetrates into the *cortex* region of the hair. This helps to temporarily add strength to the cortex. Examples include *restructurant* or protein *conditioners* and moisturising conditioners.

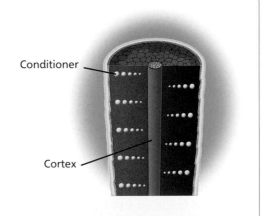

Conditioner

Cortex

Action of penetrating conditioners

Percentage of white hair – *pur-sen-tij ov wiy-t hayr* – the amount of hair on the head that is white (colourless) in comparison

candidate has shown *evidence* of performing the criteria successfully. If a candidate fails to do this, for example, not wearing personal protective equipment for Level 1 NVQ Hairdressing Standards Unit H37 *Assist with Colouring Services* PC1b, the candidate will be judged to be incompetent in that area and will be required to do the task again to gain competency.

Perm lotion – *purm lo-shun* – chemical used in the *perming* process designed to enter the *cortex* of the hair and break the *disulphide bonds* into single sulphur bonds by depositing hydrogen. Once the bonds are broken the softened hair is able to take on the shape of the *perm rod*, which is known as *moulding*. After this stage, *neutralising* is done to fix the *curl*.

Perm rods – *purm rodz* – plastic rods that come in various sizes, from small to large, which create *curls* in the hair. The length of the hair and amount of curl you want to create will determine which rods will be used. A neat section of hair the same size as the perm rod is taken and held out at 90 degrees from the head. An *end paper* is folded over the ends of the hair and the perm rod is placed in front of the end paper (facing towards the *stylist*). The ends are wound smoothly around the rod and the rod is wound towards the roots using a good amount of tension. The rod is secured by pulling the *perm rubber* over the opposite end of the perm rod.

Perm rubber – *purm rub-ur* – a stretchy rubber band attached to one end of a *perm rod*, which is used to secure the rod to the hair. It is pulled over to the opposite end of the rod once the hair has been wound onto the rod.

Perm winding – *purm wiyn-ding* – the technique used in *perming* hair by placing *perm rods* in the hair.

Permanent colour – *purm-un-unt kul-ur* – a *product* used to change the colour of hair. It consists of small *molecules* which can enter the *cortex*. *continued...*

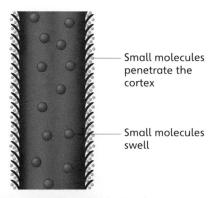

Small molecules penetrate the cortex

Small molecules swell

Effect of permanent colour on hair structure

When mixed with *hydrogen peroxide* these molecules grow in size (swell) and become trapped inside the cortex. With this type of *colouring* product the colour will have to be grown out over a period of time.

Permanent wave – *purm-un-unt way-v* – an old-fashioned term for *perming*.

Perming – *purm-ing* – the process of creating *curls* in the hair by chemically changing the hair's structure (specifically the *cortex*). There are three stages in the process: *softening*, *moulding* and *fixing*.

Permission – *pur-mi-shun* – the consent or go-ahead from someone with authority greater than one's own. See also *limit of own authority*.

Peroxide strength – *per-ox-iy-d str-eng-th* – the degree of concentration of *hydrogen peroxide* used in a *treatment*. Distilled water is added to reduce the amount of peroxide in a solution.

Personal conduct – *pur-sun-ul kon-duk-t* – the way in which a person behaves. Employees in a salon have an obligation (under *health and safety* laws) to act in a *professional* manner at all times without placing themselves and other people in the salon at *risk*.

Personal development targets – *pur-sun-ul du-vel-op-mnt tar-gitz* – see *development targets*.

Personal image – *pur-sun-ul im-ij* – the self-image created by a person, that he or she wants to project.

Personal presentation – *pur-sun-ul prez-un-tay-shun* – the appearance of a person. In hairdressing, it is important to look *professional* and to avoid wearing items which may have potential for causing accidents, such as high-heeled shoes or dangling jewellery.

Personal Protective Equipment at Work Regulations 1992 (PPE) – *pur-sun-ul pro-tek-tiv u-kwip-mnt at wurk re-gyoo-lay-shunz* – an Act which states that personal protective equipment (PPE) must be provided, maintained and used within a *workplace*. During some hairdressing treatments, especially *perming* and *relaxing* services, the *stylist* will be expected to wear appropriate protective gloves, an apron, and a face mask for mixing bleach. PPE for the client includes a gown, towels and plastic capes for protection of both skin and clothing. It is the employer's responsibility to provide PPE free of charge and to maintain it to be fit for purpose.

Personal safety – *pur-sun-ul say-f-tee* – protecting oneself from danger. It is a person's *responsibility* to act in a safe manner and avoid taking unnecessary *risks*. See also *personal space*.

Personal space – *pur-sun-ul spay-s* – the space surrounding oneself. For example, in a salon, it is important for an employee not to get too close to a client as this can make the client feel very uncomfortable or threatened; if the employee stands too far away from the client, it may appear that he or she is not interested in the client.

Personalise – *pur-sun-u-liyz* – to design something to suit someone's needs. For example, a *stylist* may need to adapt methods and techniques of *cutting* and *styling* a client's hair to fulfil a client's needs as closely as possible.

Petrissage massage – *pet-ri-sarj mas-arj* – large, circular, slow, deep kneading massage movements used to stimulate the scalp when *conditioning* hair. It increases blood flow to the area and stimulates the *sebaceous glands* to secrete *sebum*. Ultimately, it relaxes the client.

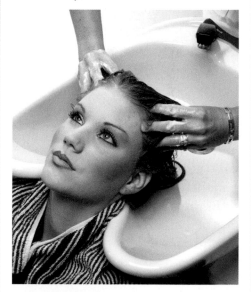

Petrissage

pH – *pee-aych* – (stands for potential of hydrogen) – a measure of how *acidic* or *alkaline* something is. If a product has the same pH as the hair and *continued...*

skin then it is said to be pH balanced and will not be harsh on the hair or scalp. It is important that products used on the scalp and hair are **compatible** with the skin's pH to avoid damage to them. See also **pH value**.

pH scale – *pee-aych skay-l* – a scale used to measure **pH**. It ranges from 1–14: 1 being highly **acidic**, 14 being highly **alkaline**. The halfway mark is 7 (neutral) and is neither acid nor alkaline. If a product is acidic its pH falls in the range of 1–6.9; if it is alkaline its pH falls in the range of 7–14. The scale is used to measure the acidity or alkalinity of cosmetic, hairdressing, household and industrial products.

pH value – *pee-aych val-yoo* – a measurement of the **pH** of something. The pH of the hair and skin is 4.5–5.5. **Semi-permanent colour** has a pH of 6.8; **permanent colour** 7.5–9.5; **bleach** 8–9.7; soap 10 and hair removal creams 11. See also **pH scale**.

Pharmacist – *far-mu-sist* – a person who is qualified and licensed to prepare and dispense drugs, including prescription drugs from a **General**

Practitioner, and non-prescription drugs which are safe to be sold over the counter.

Pheomelanin – *fee-o-mel-u-nin* – red and yellow colour **pigments** which make up the warm tones in hair.

Photographer – *fu-tog-gruf-ur* – a person **professionally** trained in taking photographs, whose services are used in hairdressing for photo shoots to demonstrate creative work and to capture images created during show and competition work.

Photographic – *fo-to-graf-ik* – produced by means of photography. For example, an **S/NVQ** candidate must supply this type of **evidence** for his or her portfolio for outcomes relating to **cutting**.

Physical change – *fiz-i-kul ch-ayn-j* – a process whereby the physical state of something changes. For example, when hair is shampooed, water is absorbed into the **cortex** of the hair and breaks down the **hydrogen bonds**. This allows the hair to be stretched. When hair is blow-dried or set, the bonds are re-formed into a new shape. This process is only temporary.

Piggyback perm wind – *pig-ee-bak purm wiyn-d* – an unconventional *perm winding* technique done by winding one *perm rod* to sit on top of the two perm rods underneath it. This produces a mixture of different *curl* sizes creating *volume* and texture in the hair.

Pigment – *pig-mnt* – the substance which colours animal tissue, such as hair and skin.

Pin – *pin* – a metal or rigid plastic clip which is pushed through a *roller* to secure the roller to the hair. Care needs to be taken not to cause any damage to the hair and scalp, or to cause any discomfort to the client.

Pin curl – *pin kur-l* – a *curl* produced by winding the hair with the fingers, rather than around a roller, and holding it in place with a *pin curl clip*. See also *pin curling*.

Pin curl clip – *pin k-url k-lip* – a two-pronged metal or plastic clip used for securing a *pin curl* to the hair. See also *pin curling*.

Pin curling – *pin k-url-ing* – a *styling* technique used when a section of hair is too small or the hair is too short to wind around a *roller*. A section of hair is taken so that it will match in with the sections taken during the rollering technique. It is then wound using one of three pin curling techniques – *flat barrel* continued...

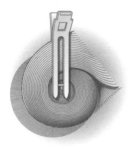

(a) Flat barrel

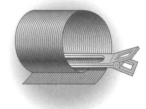

(b) Barrel

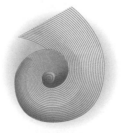

(c) Clockspring

curl, *barrel curl* or *clockspring curl* – to blend the hair in with the rest of the set. It is not suitable to do on frizzy or very long hair.

Pintail comb – *pin-tay-l ko-m* – a rigid plastic comb with a long metal end used in various aspects of hairdressing to section the hair, help **wind** hair around **rollers** or **perm rods**, or when **weaving** the hair during a **colouring** service.

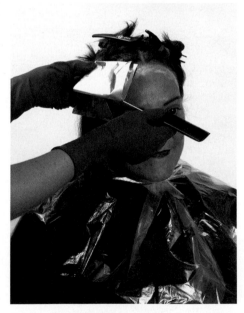

Using a pintail comb

Plait – *plat* – a length of hair made up of *intertwined* strands of hair. Formed by *plaiting*, there

are different types which produce different effects. See also **scalp plait**, **French pleat**, **corn row**.

Plaiting – *plat-ing* – a dressing technique for **styling** long hair to create **plaits**. A length of hair is sectioned, divided into strands, *intertwined* and then secured at the ends. There are many methods of plaiting from very basic to very intricate.

Plan – *p-lan* – a design or scheme laid out before an activity is performed to ensure that the activity is carried out accurately and within a set timescale.

Plasticiser – *p-last-ti-siy-zur* – a plastic resin contained in **styling** and **finishing products** which leaves a film on the hair once the hair is dry. As **atmospheric moisture** changes the internal structure of hair from **beta keratin** to **alpha keratin**, the purpose of the film is to prevent moisture from being absorbed by the hair.

Point to root – *poynt too roo-t* – a conventional drying technique that (depending on the length of the hair) will produce a looser **curl** at the roots than at the ends. It is also used in conventional *perming* techniques.

Policies – *pol-is-eez* – rules, regulations or procedures. In a *workplace*, it is essential that these are followed to ensure good practice of *health and safety*.

Porosity – *por-os-it-ee* – the ability to absorb substances.

Porosity of hair – *por-os-it-ee ov hayr* – the hair's ability to absorb *products*. The condition of the outer layer of hair (*cuticle*) determines how *porous* the hair is. If the cuticle scales are closed or lie flat, the hair will have good *porosity*; if they are tightly closed, *penetration* of products will be more difficult; if the scales are damaged and open, raised, or are missing, the hair will be over-porous and absorb chemicals too easily and quickly. See also *porosity test*.

Porosity test – *por-os-it-ee test* – a test carried out before any hairdressing *service*, to check if the *cuticle* of the hair is damaged. It is done by holding a few strands of dry hair and running the fingers from the roots to the ends and then from the ends to the roots to judge how smooth the hair feels. If it feels fairly smooth, it shows that the hair is not too *porous* and the chemical results will be even. If the hair is rough, a good end result cannot be guaranteed. A course of deep *conditioning* treatments will help the condition of the cuticle before commencing any other treatment. Also called a *texture test*.

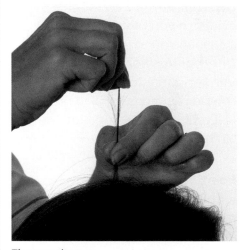

The porosity test

Porous – *por-us* – allowing the passage of liquid through something. For example, if hair is porous it will absorb water, *products* and chemicals more easily than hair that is not porous (think of how a sponge absorbs water).

103

Portfolio – *port-fo-lee-o* – a folder, either paper-based or computer-generated, in which all *evidence* is compiled, covering all competencies for the *units* that an *S/NVQ* candidate has achieved. It grows as *assessment* builds up. If the evidence is not able to be kept in the folder, such as in the case of a client's record card which needs to be retained in the salon reception, then a reference must be put in to show how the *External Verifier* can source the evidence you are claiming. Not all portfolios are checked by the *Internal Verifier* or External Verifier during a visit, but the candidate needs to keep it for reference, once completed, for up to three years.

Positive – *poz-i-tiv* – enthusiastic, effective, not *negative*. In a salon it is important to display *body language*, and respond to, and interact with, *clients* and *colleagues* in this manner.

Post-colouring treatment – *post-kul-ur-ing treet-mnt* – a *conditioner* that prevents the fading of colour in the hair. It is used after the colour has been shampooed off the hair. It closes the *cuticles*, restores the hair to its natural *pH* balance, adds moisture to the hair and helps to stop chemicals working (*creeping oxidation*).

Post-damping – *post-damp-ing* – applying *perm lotion* to the hair after it has been sectioned and wound around *perm rods*. This is the safest way of applying perm lotion and will help to ensure that all areas of the head process evenly.

Post-perm conditioner – *post-purm kon-dish-un-ur* – a special *anti-oxidant* surface conditioner used after chemical *perming* treatments to smooth the *cuticle* scales, stop chemicals working (*creeping oxidation*) and restore the hair to its natural *pH value*.

Post-relaxing treatment – *post-ru-lax-ing treet-mnt* – a cream or liquid applied to the hair after a chemical *relaxer* has been rinsed off in a *relaxing* treatment. It adds moisture to the hair and restores the hair's natural *pH* balance, counteracting the *alkalinity* of the relaxer.

Potentially harmful – *pu-ten-shul-ee harm-ful* – the possibility of being unsafe. It is important to treat and handle equipment and materials in a salon correctly. For example, if dirty scissors accidentally cut the client, it can cause *cross-infection*.

Potentially infectious condition – *pu-ten-shul-ee in-fek-shus kon-di-shun* – any *infection* or *infestation* which can be transmitted from one person to another, either by direct contact through touching, or indirectly, for example, through coughing. A common infestation found in salons is *head lice*. (See infectious diseases of the skin and scalp on pages 162–163.)

Pre-blended oil – *pree-blen-did oyl* – an oil product whose ingredients are already mixed, for example, the essential oils in an aromatherapy oil. The oil is applied to the scalp during a massage service.

Precaution – *pru-kor-shun* – taking care to avoid or prevent a dangerous or undesirable event from occurring.

Pre-colouring treatment – *pree-kul-ur-ing treet-mnt* – a *product* which evens out the

porosity of the hair before *colouring*. It helps the colour molecules to *penetrate* evenly throughout the *cortex*. Restructuring treatments will help to strengthen the internal structure of the hair.

Pre-damping – *pree-damp-ing* – applying *perm lotion* to the hair before sectioning or winding *perm rods* into the hair. This is done on *resistant hair* so that the lotion can start to soften the hair and aid winding around the rods, especially if the hair is springy. However, as there is a danger of *over-processing* the hair, this technique should be carried out quickly.

Pre-lighten – *pree-liyt-n* – to *bleach* the hair when the required amount of lift cannot be achieved using *permanent colour* or a *high-lift tint*, for example, if a client has a base 3 hair colour and wants to achieve a target colour of a base 8 with a red tone. A permanent tint can only achieve three levels of lift, so the hair will be pre-lightened to the degree required and then the target colour would be applied over the top. It is important to observe a bleaching product constantly as it will react differently on continued...

different hair types; if you exceed the levels of lift you require, the target colour will not be achievable.

Pre-locking stage – *pree-lok-ing st-ayj* – the preparation of the hair before *locking* is carried out.

Preparation – *prep-ur-ay-shun* – the putting together beforehand of all the materials and equipment that are required to complete a *service*. For example, for a *colouring* service, a shade chart to choose the colour with the client, bowls for mixing, combs and clips for sectioning are all needed.

Pre-perm treatment – *pree-purm treet-mnt* – a specialist *product* applied before *perming* to even out the *porosity* of the *hair* along the *hair shaft*. This will help to ensure an even *curl* throughout the hair's *length*. If it is not used when the hair is porous, an uneven curl formation (tighter ends and looser roots) or *frizziness* will occur.

Pre-pigmentation – *pree-pig-mun-tay-shun* – the term used for restoring or adding missing *warm tones* (gold, copper, red) to hair, previously removed as a result of lightening processes or the use of a colour remover. The process ensures that the *target colour* will be achieved and warm tones in the hair will be maintained when colouring the hair darker. It can be done by using *temporary colour*, *semi-permanent colour*, *quasi-permanent* or *permanent colour* products.

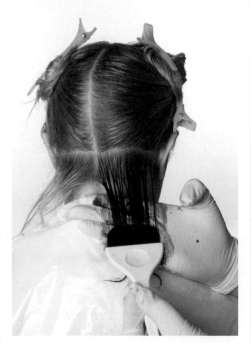

Applying missing copper tone to hair

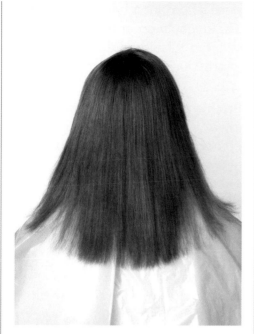

Hair after pigmentation and before applying permanent colour

following the **manufacturer's instructions**. It is then removed with dry cotton wool and the result is **assessed** to determine if the full **treatment** can be carried out.

Pre-relaxing treatment – *pree-ru-lax-ing treet-mnt* – a **treatment** used on dry or porous hair before chemically relaxing the hair. It coats the **cuticle** with a film which acts as a barrier, thereby slowing down the action of the chemicals that will be applied during the **relaxing treatment**. This prevents **over-processing** and maintains the **condition** of the hair.

Pre-relaxer test – *pree-ru-lax-ur test* – a test to determine whether a **product** for a **relaxing treatment** is suitable to use on a client's hair and to determine the speed at which the natural **curl** will be removed. It is also useful to perform if the history and condition of the client's hair is unknown. A small section of hair is sectioned away from the rest of the hair, using aluminium foil placed as close as possible to the scalp. The chosen strength of relaxer is applied to the strand of hair and allowed to process

Pre-softening – *pree-sof-ning* – the method of applying a weak **hydrogen peroxide** solution to the hair to lift and swell the **cuticles**. This allows chemical **colouring** products to **penetrate resistant hair**.

Pressing comb – *pres-ing ko-m* – a heated tool used during **thermal styling** to straighten the hair temporarily.

Pressing technique – *pres-ing tek-neek* – a way of temporarily straightening hair using a **pressing comb**.

Previous records – *pree-vy-us rek-ords* – the recorded history of something or someone. A **client record** gives the hair **service** history of the client and can describe, for example, any **negative reactions** which have taken place, the client's preferred hair colours and any other **treatment** considerations that need to be taken into account.

Price – *pr-iy-s* – the cost of a **service** or **product**. It may vary from salon to salon and area to area. A price list should be displayed in full view, both to inform a client and as a form of advertising.

Price structure – *pr-iy-s struk-chur* – the charges and policies connected with charges. In a salon, these should be clearly set out in a price list and be competitive with other salons in the area. It should also state methods of payment, such as cash only, or no credit given, and any requirements for a deposit on a treatment, which may be non-refundable. A clearly written policy means that both staff and customers fully understand the ground rules for payment.

Prices Act 1974 – *pr-iy-sez akt* – an Act which stipulates that the price of products has to be clearly displayed, in order to prevent giving a false or misleading impression to the buyer or client.

Prickle cell layer – *pri-kul sel lay-ur* – the fourth layer of the **epidermis** within the skin, found between the **granular layer** above it and the **basal layer** below it. It is the layer in which living cells begin changing into **keratin**. The cells are shaped like spikes, which allows them to attach to other cells. (See the structure of the skin diagram on page 159.)

Primary colours – *pr-iy-mur-ee kul-urz* – the colours red, yellow and blue, found on a **colour wheel**. They are used to make the **secondary tones**.

Primary tone – *pr-iy-mur-ee tow-n* – different from a **primary colour**, it indicates how warm or cool a colour is. There are six main tones that are given numbers on colour charts to help a hairdresser to identify what the primary and secondary tones in the colours are: 1 = ash; 2 = mauve; 3 = gold; 4 = red; 5 = mahogany; 6 = violet; 7 = brunette; 8 = pearl. These tones change according to manufacturer.

The first number on a colour chart is the basic hair colour, indicating how dark or light the colour is. The first number after the decimal point or slash is the primary tone (the strongest tone) and the second number after the decimal point or slash is the *secondary tone*. So, for example, on a *permanent colour* chart the number 8.34 (8/34) indicates that the *base colour* is light blonde (see *depth*), the primary tone is gold and the secondary tone is red. See also *international colour chart*.

Procedure – *pro-see-jur* – a process or system for doing things in a certain way.

Product – *pro-duk-t* –
1. *products for sale*, such as retail goods for home use in a salon (e.g. shampoos and conditioners);
2. *stock* used within a hairdressing *service*, such as *colouring* products, *finishing products* and so on.

Product display – *pro-duk-t dis-pl-ay* – a presentation of retail products available for sale. They are often attractively arranged within the reception area to encourage clients to buy them.

Product knowledge – *pro-duk-t no-lij* – the information a person has about a *product*. Knowing the benefits and features of each item of stock, such as its ingredients, application advice and correct storage, helps to sell the product to a client.

Productive – *pro-duk-tiv* – creative, fruitful, showing good results from effort.

Productivity – *pro-duk-tiv-it-ee* – the production or output of something.

Productivity target – *pro-duk-tiv-it-ee tar-git* – a goal to achieve a certain level of output or income, such as the number of hairdressing *services* delivered, or the amount of income from retail *sales*.

Products for sale – *pro-duk-ts for say-l* – retail *products* for sale to clients for home use, often used to *complement* the products used within a *service*. See also *product display*.

Professional – *pro-fesh-un-ul* – expert, skilful or proficient in a particular field, through *training* and practice.

Profit – *pro-fit* – the amount of money left over in a business after the deduction of bills, outgoings and wages. If outgoings in a salon are greater than money coming in, there is no profit to reinvest and the salon will eventually go out of business.

Project – *pro-jek-t* – a task usually referring to one done as part of an **S/NVQ** course of study. It is set by a tutor or an **assessor** and has set **objectives** with requirements that need to be met.

Promotional activity – *pro-mo-shun-ul ak-tiv-i-tee* – an event whose aim is to publicise a **product** or **service** for a business. Forms of media used to promote this are television, radio, national and local newspaper advertisements, websites, leaflets or fliers.

Promotions – *pro-mo-shuns* – raising the public's awareness of products, services and activities. For example, a salon may decide to advertise seasonal special offers or run a **promotional activity** to publicise new trends in hairstyles.

Proportion – *pro-por-shun* – the comparative relationship of parts to the whole. For example, *hair extensions* need to look well-proportioned in relation to a **client's features**.

Protection – *pro-tek-shun* – defence or safeguarding. For example, in the skin **keratin** makes skin hard and difficult to **penetrate**, **nerve endings** provide early detection of possible skin problems, the **subcutaneous layer** protects internal organs, and the **acid mantle** helps prevent **bacteria** from entering the skin.

Provision and Use of Work Equipment Regulations 1998 – *prov-i-shun nd yoos ov wurk u-kwip-mnt reg-yoo-lay-shunz* – these regulations require the **employer** to prevent and control the **risks** to **employees' health and safety** when using **equipment** within the **workplace**. The equipment must be suitable for use, regularly maintained, inspected regularly and used only by people trained in the correct use, following the manufacturer's guidelines.

Psoriasis – *sor-iy-a-sis* – a skin **condition** recognised by red thickened skin covered with dry, silvery, scaly patches. It is commonly found along the hairline, behind the ears, and on the knees and elbows. It can be itchy and bleed when scratched, risking *infection* at the site. It is thought to be a result of higher than normal production and shedding of the *epidermis* cells. It may be made worse by stress, but responds favourably to sunlight or ultra-violet radiation from sun beds. A *medical referral* to a *general practitioner* is recommended.

Purchases – *pur-chu-siz* – items or *stock* bought.

Pus – *pus* – a thick yellowish or green fluid, produced as a result of *infection*. It is made up of serum, tissue fragments, dead *bacteria* and white *blood* cells and varies in odour and consistency.

Pustule – *pus-tyoo-l* – a small, round, raised area of skin which contains *pus*, such as the lesions found in *acne*, *eczema*, *impetigo* and other *infections*. (See infectious diseases of the skin and scalp on pages 162–163.)

Qualification – *kwal–if-i-kay-shun* – an award gained for the completion of a course. In an *S/NVQ* hairdressing course, once all *units* are completed and all *Performance Criteria* and *ranges* have been covered and assessed, the candidate will be awarded a certificate showing that he or she has worked to complete the standards set by the *Awarding Body*. See also *National Vocational Qualification*.

Qualification framework – *kwal-if-i-kay-shun fraym-wurk* – a combination of *National Vocational Qualification* (NVQ) units taken from existing NVQs arranged to form the basis of a *qualification* in a field of study which best matches the needs of a candidate or an employer.

Quasi–permanent colour – *kway-ziy-pur-mun-unt kul-ur* – a thick liquid-based *product* mixed with a weak *developer* used to colour hair. It has smaller *molecules* than *permanent colour* which enter the *cortex*, but it does not change hair colour permanently or lighten hair. It covers a high *percentage of white hair*. It may leave a *re-growth* when used over a period of time because of the developer used in mixing the colour.

Question – *kwes-chun* – a query requiring an answer. See also *open questions* and *closed questions*.

Race Relations Act 1976 (amended 2000) – *ray-s ru-lay-shunz akt* – an Act which states that it is unlawful to discriminate against a person in employment regardless of that person's race, colour, nationality, or ethnic origin. A policy of equal opportunities must be in place otherwise a business could be liable to prosecution if a person feels harassed or discriminated against because of their race.

Radiotherapy – *ray-dee-o-ther-u-pee* – a medical treatment for *disease*, especially of cancer, using radioactive substances. This medical treatment is a *contraindication* to some scalp massage techniques, such as *high frequency* treatments. See also *chemotherapy*.

Range – *rayn-j* – a variety of situations within a course of study for which an *S/NVQ* candidate must show competence in knowledge and performance. In hairdressing, examples include the use of *products* and techniques and administering tests. It also applies to the candidate's *appearance*, personal conduct, personal hygiene, reliability, punctuality and the ability to work with others in a team.

Razor – *ray-zur* – a tool with a sharp blade used to cut hair (see *razoring*) or to remove facial hair during a *shaving* service. Disposable blades are often used for *health and safety* reasons to avoid *cross-infection*, in case the skin is accidentally cut. They should always be used on wet hair as *cutting* dry hair with a razor can cause pain.

Razoring – *ray-zur-ing* – using a *razor* to cut hair. The method is done to remove *length* and bulk or to thin out the ends of hair. A section of hair is taken and the razor is placed adjacent (across) to it. The hair is cut by sliding the razor along the hair shaft (not too close to the roots) with smooth strokes, moving from the wrist.

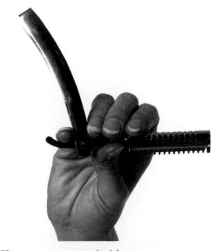

The correct way to hold a razor

113

Realistic working environment (RWE) – *ree-u-lis-tik wur-king en-vy-ron-mnt* – an environment which reflects a real work situation. In order to meet *NOS* client specifications, *assessment* centres for hairdressing must duplicate what takes place within a commercial salon and include sales and marketing policies which attract a variety of clients.

Reassure – *ree-a-shor* – to restore confidence or set one's mind at rest, for example, setting a client's mind at rest that the products being sold are the correct ones for the client.

Receipt – *ru-see-t* – an acknowledgement of payment, which holds all the information relating to the purchase. This may be required when a client returns goods to a salon. See also *Sale of Goods Act 1994*.

Reception – *ru-sep-shun* – the area at the front of a salon where *appointments* are made and which the client first sees when entering the salon. *Responsibilities* in this area include *maintenance*, keeping it clean and tidy at all times, welcoming and attending to clients' and telephone enquiries, making appointments for salon *services* and handling payments from clients.

Recommendation – *rek-om-end-ay-shun* – a suggestion appropriate to someone's needs. This could be advising a client on an appropriate *service* or *product*, based on *client needs* and *analysis* of the client's scalp and hair. This can be noted on the *client record* for future reference. See also *necessary tests*.

Record keeping – *rek-ord kee-ping* – a method of storing *confidential* details about a client, which can be stored in a locked cabinet or on a computer. See also *client record* and *Data Protection Act 1998*.

Record of achievement – *rek-ord ov a-cheev-mnt* – a record, at the front of an *S/NVQ* candidate's *assessment* book, which is filled in as each *unit* is completed. Once an *assessor* is satisfied with the unit *evidence*, showing *ranges* and *knowledge* covered, and all *portfolio* work in place, he or she will sign off the unit with a signature and date. Once all the units have been completed the relevant *qualification* can be applied for.

Recording – *ruk-or-ding* – making copies or notes of conversations or events that have taken place to store. Once this information is stored it can be used at a later date, if necessary.

Reduce degree of curl – *ru-joos du-gree ov kur-l* – to reduce the amount of **curl** in hair, for example, by **relaxing** the hair.

Reduction – *ru-duk-shun* – a process by which the addition of hydrogen **reduces** the amount of oxygen (opposite of **oxidation**). Lifting colour from hair by using a colour reducer is an example of this process.

Refer – *ru-fur* – to transfer or pass on, to recommend. It is important to guide someone to the most appropriate person to provide the correct information. See also **medical referral**.

Reflective account – *ru-flek-tiv ak-ownt* – an explanation of a process of work undertaken by an **S/NVQ** candidate either in written form or as a case study, which includes the candidate's personal reflections of the situation. It is signed by the candidate, the **assessor** and the client. If done

orally, the candidate talks through the choices made in relation to the client's needs, such as reasons for any products chosen, and aftercare **recommendations**, and the discussion is logged in the candidate's **assessment** book.

Re-growth – *ree-grow-th* – a band of new hair growth at the roots that is different in colour from the rest of the hair. This occurs when a **permanent colour** has started to grow out.

Re-growth application – *ree-grow-th ap-li-kay-shun* – applying colour to a **re-growth** area. See also **banding**.

Regular – *reg-yoo-lur* – occurring repeatedly, such as a client who often comes to the salon. The **client record** will need to be updated at each visit.

Relax – *ru-lax* – to **reduce** or straighten the natural **curl** in hair.

Relaxing product – *ru-lax-ing prod-uk-t* – a highly **alkaline** product used to chemically **relax** naturally curly hair. It opens and swells the **cuticle** so that *continued...*

115

it can enter the **cortex**. Once in the cortex it breaks down some of the **disulphide bonds** and the hair is straightened using a comb or the fingers. As the hair straightens, a new amino acid called lanthionine is formed. Once the hair is sufficiently straightened, the lanthionine is removed by rinsing. **Neutralising shampoo** is then applied to fix the hair in its new style. Often called **relaxer**.

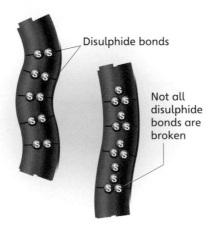

Disulphide bonds

Not all disulphide bonds are broken

How relaxing products work

Relevant person – *rel-u-vunt pur-sun* – the person responsible for a particular **job role** or a specific area of expertise.

Relevant rights – *rel-u-vunt riyts* – the rights relevant to a person, such as those for clients listed under various **legislation** Acts. (See legislation on pages 164–165.)

Remedial action – *ru-meed-ee-ul ak-shun* – action taken to remedy or fix a problem, for example, immediately rinsing off **perm lotion** if a client complains of a severe burning sensation.

Remove curl – *ru-moov kur-l* – to take away **curl** in the hair. A **relaxing** process makes the hair straight.

Reporting of Injuries, Diseases & Dangerous Occurrences Regulations 1995 (RIDDOR) – *ru-por-ting ov in-jur-eez diz-eez-iz nd dayn-jur-us o-kur-un-sez reg-yoo-lay-shunz* – these regulations state that all accidents must be reported and, in some circumstances, must be reported to the local environmental health officer.

Reporting problems – *ru-por-ting prob-lums* – telling the **relevant person** in a workplace a problem which has occurred, or a risk which is likely to affect salon **services**. There may be a particular **procedure** to follow.

Resale Prices Act 1964 and 1976 – *ree-say-l pr-iy-sez akt* – these Acts state that although manufacturers can supply products at the recommended price, the seller is not obliged to sell them at it. A seller must ensure that the products are of satisfactory quality, and that they are fit for their stated purpose.

Resistant hair – *ru-zis-tnt hayr* – hair that has a thick, tightly compacted **cuticle**, or is coated with **products**, making it difficult for chemical processes to enter the **cortex**. For example, Oriental hair, grey/white hair, or coarse hair has more layers of cuticle than European or African Caribbean hair so does not easily allow the products to **penetrate** into the cortex and develop.

Resolve – *ru-zol-v* – to solve a problem, or sort out a disagreement, either informally with colleagues in a helpful way, or more formally through a **grievance procedure**.

Resources – *ru-zor-sez* – assets of a business or elements which generate income or are required to perform a hair **service**, such as electricity, water, gas and so on.

Responsibility – *rus-pon-su-bil-it-ee* – a duty, task or decision someone has to do or make.

Responsible person – *rus-pon-si-bul pur-sun* – the person in charge of carrying out, or overseeing, a task. For example, a supervisor, line manager or employer is responsible for **health and safety** issues, such as identifying and **controlling risks**.

Restore depth and tone – *ru-stor dep-th nd tow-n* – to bring back **depth** and brightness to hair colour, by re-colouring the hair. For example, when the tone of the colour, for example, red or copper, is not as vibrant as when the hair was first coloured.

Restore pH balance – *ru-stor pee-aych bal-uns* – to return the **pH** balance of the hair back to its natural pH (4.5–5.5) after **perming**, **relaxing**, **colouring** and **bleaching**. pH-balanced conditioners are used to do this.

Restriction – *ru-strik-shun* – a limitation. For example, if a client's hair has poor **elasticity** from **over-processing** it will restrict the use of further continued...

chemical treatments due to the risk of hair breakage.

Restructurant – *ree-struk-chur-unt* – a *conditioning* product applied to hair which has been damaged, to protect the hair from any further damage. See also *pre-colouring treatment*, *pre-perm treatment*.

Restyle – *ree-stiyl* – a significant change in the weight, length, shape, style or volume of a client's hairstyle.

Review – *ru-v-yoo* – to check or go over something, to evaluate and consider options. An *S/NVQ* candidate may do this regularly with an assessor or tutor.

Ringworm – *ring-w-urm* – a *fungal* skin *infection*, initially seen as small round, red spots, growing into larger spots with a raised scaly border. It often causes hair to fall out, creating bald patches. It occurs in the beard area and other areas of the body. It is highly infectious and should not be treated in the salon. A *medical referral* should be recommended. Also known as *tinea*. (See infectious diseases of the skin and scalp on pages 162–163.)

Risk – *ri-sk* – a danger or *hazard*. Preventative measures need to be put in place to reduce the number of *potentially harmful* situations developing in a salon.

Risk assessment – *ri-sk u-ses-mnt* – a careful examination of potential *hazards* to people's *health and safety* which could occur in the workplace. This is done to *assess* whether it is possible to prevent accidents occurring. It involves: identifying the hazard; deciding who might be harmed and how; evaluating the risk and deciding on precautions to take; recording and implementing any necessary policies or procedures; reviewing the assessment and updating it when necessary.

Role – *r-ol* – the duty, job or *responsibility* that a person is assigned or takes on.

Roller – *r-ol-ur* – a plastic cylinder (tube shape), used in *perming* and *setting*, around which hair is wound to form a *curl*. It comes in a variety of sizes; the length of the hair and the degree of curl required determines the size of the roller used.

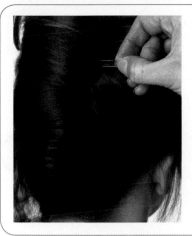

Rolls – *r-ols* – a dressing technique for *styling* long hair in which hair is rolled up in a cylindrical form. Rolls can be used anywhere on the head depending on the effect to be achieved. The most common form is a **vertical roll** or **French pleat**. The size and position of the roll can be adapted to produce different fashion effects.

Securing a vertical roll (French pleat)

Root drag – *root drag* – when hair is lifted away from the head at an angle less than or greater than 90 degrees from the root area. This can be purposely done to create styles where the curl needs to sit flatter on the head.

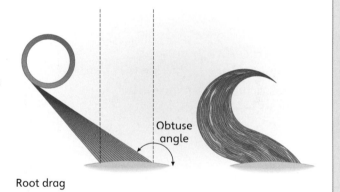

Obtuse angle

Root drag

Root lift – *root-lift* – the lifting of hair upwards and away from the root area to give body and height to a style; winding **rollers** and **perm rods**, so that each section of hair, suitable for the size of the roller/rod, sits on its own base to create maximum root lift.

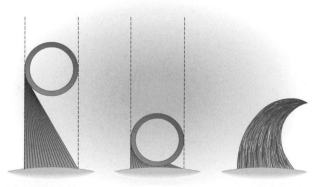

Root lift

119

Root perm winding – *r-oot purm wiyn-ding* – an unconventional form of **perm winding** whereby **perm rods** are placed at mid-lengths of hair and wound down to the roots. This creates **root lift** rather than curly ends. Also called **root wind**.

Root to point winding – *r-oot too poynt wiyn-ding* – a **winding technique** used in both **setting** and **perm winding** whereby the hair is wound around a **roller** or **perm rod** in a spiral manner to produce a **curl** with an even diameter throughout. A better result is achieved on shoulder length or long hair.

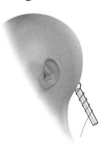

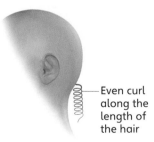

Even curl along the length of the hair

Root to point winding

Rotary massage – *ro-tur-ee mas-arj* – small, firm, circular massage movements using the pads of the fingers to massage **shampoo** into the hair and scalp, and to remove dirt, products and **sebum**.

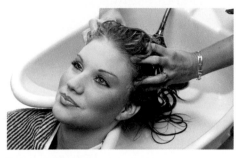

Rotary massage

Rough dry – *r-uf driy* – to remove excess moisture from the hair, with a towel or blow-dryer, before using **styling** tools or **equipment**. Doing this first before a **blow-drying** service avoids putting extra tension, and causing wear and tear, on wet hair. The process also helps to create **root lift**.

Round brush – *row-nd br-ush* – a round bristle brush that comes in a variety of shapes and sizes to suit different lengths and textures of hair. A **mesh of hair** is wound around the brush and dried so that the hair takes on the shape of the brush. It is also used to create **root lift** and flicks in the hair.

Round face shape – *row-nd fay-s shay-p* – the **head and face shape** determined by a short and broad face with full cheeks and round contours. Width at the top of the head should be provided with height from the hair, which should be worn close at the sides, so that the round face is made to look as oval as possible. Ensuring lots of height and softness in the fringe area, such as a half **fringe** with soft tendrils to hide the roundness of the jaw line, is important for this shape.

Rounded neckline – *row-n-did nek-liyn* – the shape determined by **cutting** a rounded outline at the **nape** of the neck in which the corners are removed to create a soft rounded shape. Unwanted hair is removed from outside the neckline shape to produce a clean, accurately rounded end result.

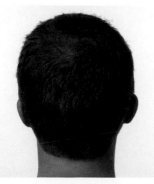

Rounded neckline

Rubber band marks – *rub-ur ban-d mar-ks* – hair damage caused by **perm rubbers**.

121

Safe working practice – *say-f wurk-ing prak-tis* – the practice of taking all possible steps to ensure the **health and safety** of people in a **workplace**. For example, ensuring an **employee** uses **equipment** according to **manufacturer's instructions**, partakes in full safety training, conducts good relationships with **colleagues** and clients, and fulfils his or her **responsibilities** in a **professional** manner.

Safeguard – *say-f-gar-d* – to protect against harm or danger, especially in the workplace. See also **Control of Substances Hazardous to Health Regulations 2002**, **Health and Safety at Work Act 1974**.

Safety razor – *say-f-tee ray-zur* – see **disposable blade razor**.

Sale of Goods Act 1979 and 1995 / Supply of Goods and Services Act 1982 – *sayl ov gudz akt nd sup-liy ov gudz nd sur-vis-ez akt* – as a hairdresser, this Act means that all the treatments given to a client must be as stated in the service agreement or price list and should be carried out within a commercially acceptable time.

Sale and Supply of Goods Act 1994 – *sayl nd sup-liy ov gudz akt* – this Act states that:

Goods must be:

- of merchantable quality
- fit for the purpose for which they are sold
- as described in their advertising.

Services must be:

- charged at a reasonable price
- provided within a reasonable time
- given with reasonable care and skill.

Sales – *sayl-z* – the action of **selling**. A large part of a salon's business is through promoting the buying of **products** and **services**.

Salon activities – *sal-on ak-tiv-it-eez* – activities carried out by a salon to generate immediate and future income for the business, such as **promotional activities** for new **products** and/or **services**, or training **employees** to learn new techniques or discover the latest trends in hairdressing.

Salon requirements – *sal-on ru-kwiyr-mnts* – rules, regulations and principles set up within a salon to cover all aspects of **health and safety**, data protection, **equal opportunities**, disability discrimination, **legislation** and regulation of **products** and **services**. (See legislation on pages 164–165.)

Salon services – *sal-on sur-vi-sez* – all **services** offered within a salon, including **consultation** and practical **treatments**, **advice** and aftercare.

Salon standards – *sal-on stan-dudz* – rules in a salon related to employees' **appearance** and behaviour, **services** carried out, **job roles** and management structuring, **policies** in dealing with complaints, and **health and safety** practices. (See legislation on pages 164–165.)

Salon time – *sa-lon tiy-m* – the time spent in a **professional** capacity with clients within a salon. It excludes down time or relaxation time.

Scabies – *scay-beez* – a skin **disease** in which red irritating spots and lines appear, the result of the itch mite **parasite** boring beneath the skin. It causes intense itching to the sufferer. It is highly

contagious and a referral needs to be recommended to a **General Practitioner**. (See infectious diseases of the skin and scalp on pages 162–163.)

Scalp – *scal-p* – the skin that covers the bones of the skull.

Scalp irritation – *scal-p i-rit-ay-shun* – itchiness, soreness, redness or **inflammation** of the scalp experienced by a client especially if the client is sensitive to a hairdressing **product**. Cuts or abrasions on the scalp may indicate a **contraindication** to certain hairdressing **services** such as **colouring** or **perming**.

Scalp plait – *scal-p plat* – a traditional **plait** that sits *continued...*

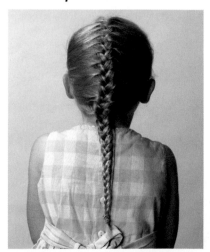

A scalp plait

close to the scalp. It is a dressing technique used for **styling** long hair which involves alternately crossing three strands of hair over one another until all the hair on the head is incorporated into the plait. Also called **French plait**.

Scalp treatments – *scal-p treet-mnts* – **products** applied to the scalp to either moisturise and nourish a dry scalp or promote hair growth. For example, olive oil can be warmed and applied, massaged and removed with an initial application of neat **shampoo**. Once all the oil is removed use shampoo and **conditioner** as normal.

Scar tissue – *scar tish-yoo* – new skin which has formed to cover a break in the skin. Recent scar tissue is a **contraindication** to some scalp massage techniques, such as **high frequency** services. Older, completely healed scar tissue is not normally classed as a contraindication. If in doubt, check with the salon manager.

Scarlet fever – *scar-lut fee-vur* – a bacterial **infection**, found mainly in children, starting with a sore throat, fever and an eruption of a scarlet rash on the skin – hence

the name. It is **contagious** and is a **notifiable** disease.

Scheduling – *shed-yoo-ling* – fitting in and rearranging appointments to gain maximum **productivity** time and avoid having long periods of inactivity in a salon working day.

Scissor-over-comb – *siz-ur o-vur ko-m* – a **cutting** method used with only **scissors** and a **cutting comb**, ideal for hair that is too short to hold, for **tapering** hair into the hairline or neck or for getting in difficult to reach areas. It is used to cut hair very short. It is commonly used in the **nape** area and around the ears following the natural contours of the head.

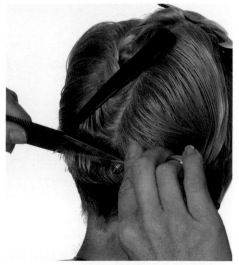

Scissor-over-comb technique

Scissors – *siz-urz* – a tool with sharp blades fastened in the middle, used for *cutting* hair. They are the most important piece of *equipment* for a *stylist*, varying in design, size and price. Examples include off-set scissors, on which the thumb hold is set higher than the finger hold for comfort; scissors with plain, *serrated*, long or short blades; light or heavy scissors; training scissors, which are cheaper because they are often dropped; and scissors high in price because of the quality of the metal and their precision for cutting.

Scope and responsibility – *sko-p nd rus-pon-si-bi-li-tee* – the limits of *responsibility* a person has, particularly in relation to *health and safety*, according to his or her *training* and *job role*.

Scrunch dry – *s-krun-ch driy* – see *finger dry*.

Sculptured – *skul-p-chud* – hair that has been modelled into three-dimensional shapes.

Sebaceous glands – *se-bay-shus g-lands* – *glands* found in the *dermis* of the skin, situated next to *hair follicles*. They secrete *sebum* and, when mixed with sweat, form the *acid mantle* on the skin, which offers *protection* against *micro-organisms* and *infection*. Over-production of sebum caused by stimulation, *hormone* imbalance or illness results in oily skin and scalp, giving the hair a greasy look and feel. Under-production of sebum may leave the skin and scalp dry and cracked, with visible flakes. There are no sebaceous glands on the palms of the hands or the soles of the feet, as there are no hair follicle openings in these areas. (See the structure of the skin diagram on page 159.)

Seborrhoea – *seb-o-ree-uh* – oily skin caused by overactive *sebaceous glands*, especially on the face, scalp, chest and back. It is more common in males because of the influence of male *hormones*, so it is most commonly found in adolescent males, whose hormone levels are unstable. It can lead to skin congestion and *acne*.

Sebum – *see-bm* – a mixture of fatty acids and cholesterol (an important component of cell *membranes* and needed for producing *hormones*) produced by the *sebaceous glands* and secreted onto the skin's *continued…*

surface to help keep the skin moist. Together with sweat it forms the **acid mantle**. (See the structure of the skin diagram on page 159.)

Secondary colours – sek-on-dur-ee kul-urz – the colours orange, green and violet, made from mixing the **primary colours** and which form part of the **colour wheel**.

Secondary tone – sek-on-dur-ee tow-n – a tone which is weaker in intensity than the **primary tone** of a colour. On a colour chart it is denoted by the second number after the decimal point or slash.

Secrete – se-kreet – to produce and release a substance, such as **glands** releasing **hormones** in the body.

Section marks – sek-shun mar-ks – marks, gaps or divisions which are left in the hair after the hair has been dried around a roller and the roller has been taken out. It can also be created by **perm rods** during a **perming** service. These can be removed by **teasing**, **backcombing** or **backbrushing**.

Sectioning clips – sek-shun-ing kli-ps – clips used to divide or section off large quantities of hair and hold the hair in place. They allow a **stylist** to cut hair in a methodical way and to work with hair more precisely, such as when **nine section perm winding** and **colouring**.

Secure – se-kyoor – to fasten firmly. Hair grips, **pins**, bands and so on are used to ensure the hair stays in place, for example, when a **stylist** pins a **French pleat** in place to avoid it falling down during **competition work**.

Security procedures – se-kyoor-itee pru-see-jur-z – rules that need to be followed to make a business premises secure from criminal damage. Examples include ways to handle money deposits, and protecting a salon from theft.

Seepage – seep-ij – when a **product** escapes from its package (mesh, foil, etc.) as a result of the mixture being too runny, or from too much heat being applied. This may cause a patchy result at the roots where the colour has leaked.

Self-employed – sel-f em-ploy-d – working for oneself on a freelance basis rather than for an *employer*. Often a *stylist* will rent chair space in a salon and contribute towards the running costs of the salon. This type of worker is responsible for managing his or her own tax payments and *insurance* contributions.

Selling – *sel-ing* – putting something up for sale, or encouraging a buyer to give money in exchange for something. For example, to introduce a client to the *products* or *services* most suitable for the client, it is important for a salon *employee* to have full knowledge of each. See also *benefits of products*.

Semi-permanent colour – *sem-ee-purm-un-unt kul-ur* – a liquid-based *colouring* product, applied to wet hair (previously

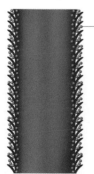

Small molecules penetrate into the cuticle and outer edge of the cortex

Effect of semi-permanent colour on hair structure

shampooed) to colour the hair. It has a mixture of large and small *molecules* that *penetrate* the *cuticle*, some penetrating the outer layer of the *cortex*. It lasts from 4 to 8 *shampoos* and covers up to 30% of *white hair*. It does not have the ability to lighten the hair.

Senegalese twist – *sen-a-gul-eez tw-ist* – a method of creating intricate patterns in the hair, originating from Senegal, Africa.

Sensation – *sen-say-shun* – the feeling that occurs when the skin makes contact with something. It is perceived by the *nerve endings* in the skin and helps the body to protect itself from harm, such as avoiding touching very hot items.

Sensitised hair – *sen-sit-iyzd hayr* – hair that has been made more sensitive or *porous* than normal due to the use of chemical products such as *bleaching*. The hair will need to be treated carefully as it can break easily.

Sequencing – *see-kwn-sing* – the ordering of one or more steps so that they follow each *continued...*

other logically or methodically, are cost-effective and make efficient use of time.

Serrated – *sur-ayt-id* – having a saw-like edge. See also *thinning scissors*.

Serrated scissors – *sur-ayt-id siz-urz* – see *thinning scissors*.

Services – *sur-vis-ez* – the range of physical and chemical *treatments* which a salon offers to clients in return for payment.

Setting – *set-ing* – a process that enables straight hair to be made curly and curly hair to be made straighter. After hair is divided into sections to suit the size of the *rollers*, it is wound around the rollers and then dried using added heat to fix the *curl*. If heated rollers are being used, dry hair is allowed to cool around the rollers to fix the curl. The hair's structure allows this process to take place by the breaking down and re-forming of the *hydrogen bonds*. See also *alpha keratin* and *beta keratin*.

Setting aids – *set-ing ay-dz* – see *styling aids*.

Sew – *so* – to join or decorate with a needle and thread, for example, *hair extensions* are sewn into natural hair.

Sex Discrimination Act 1975 and 1986 – *sex dis-krim-in-ay-shun akt* – this Act states that it is unlawful to discriminate between men and women in relation to job opportunities, pay and marital status.

Shampoo – *sham-poo* – a *product* applied to the hair to cleanse and remove dirt and natural grease (*sebum*). See also *clarifying shampoo*.

Shampoo massage techniques – *sham-poo mas-arj tek-neeks* – the massage movements used to shampoo hair, such as *effleurage massage*, *rotary massage*, *friction massage*.

Shape – *shay-p* – an outline, such as the shape of a hairstyle. It should look even and balanced, and *complement* the face shape of the client. (See head and face shapes on page 161.)

Shaving – *shay-ving* – see *shaving service*.

Shaving service – *shay-ving sur-vis* – a *service* that removes hair from the face to produce a clean shaven look, with a smooth feel to the skin.

Shaving techniques – *shay-ving tek-neeks* – the wet or dry techniques carried out during a *shaving service*. Dry shaving involves using an electric shaver which may be powered by batteries or mains electricity. In wet shaving the area is prepared by using a *lathering product*. The hair is then removed with a *razor* while the hair is still wet using a *cut-throat razor* or *safety razor*.

Shine spray – *shiy-n sp-ray* – a *finishing product* designed to give the hair maximum shine, used in the same way as hairspray. It leaves a coating of shiny residue on the hair to create sheen.

Short graduation – *sh-ort grad-yoo-ay-shun* – when the inner layers of the hair *lengths* are longer than the outline shape (perimeter edge) of a haircut. See also *long graduation*.

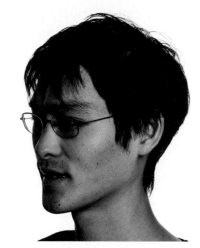

A short graduated haircut showing longer length at the top of the head

Shortage – *shor-tij* – the difference between what there should be and what there actually is. For example, there may be a shortfall of money in the till, because of incorrect change having been given.

Show audience – *sho or-dee-uns* – spectators who come to watch a hairdressing show or competition.

Sideburns – *siyd-burns* – facial hair growing down both sides of the face in front of the ears and on the cheeks of male clients. These can be cut and shaped using *scissor-over-comb* or *clipper-over-comb* continued...

129

cutting methods. The length of the hair at the sides of the head is used as a guide to ensure they are blended into the rest of the style. They are balanced on both sides of the head by using the edge of the clippers flat to the head, creating a clean sharp line. The outline shape may require *shaving* once the cut is completed.

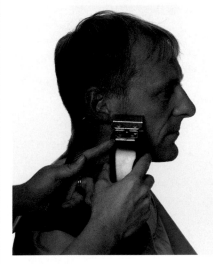

Shaping sideburns

Silky locks – *sil-kee lox* – synthetic or human hair which is wrapped around natural braided hair.

Simulation – *sim-yoo-lay-shun* – the imitation of the conditions which reflect a real situation. It is sometimes carried out during *training* when the real situation does not occur frequently or when it would be inappropriate to carry it out, such as a role play activity in which an **employee** has to learn to deal with an angry client. A fire evacuation drill is another example.

Single action perm – *sin-gul ak-shun purm* – a **perm lotion** containing the active chemical ammonium thioglycollate of which only one application is applied to African Caribbean hair during the **perming** process. Developed for African Caribbean hair, it stops the hair from becoming chemically damaged. The perm remains on the hair throughout the process (during **smoothing** and **straightening** and when the hair is wound around the **perm rods**).

Skills for life – *skilz fur liyf* – see *basic skills*.

Skin – *skin* – the largest organ of the body which is the external covering of the body. It varies in thickness, being toughest on the soles of the feet and thinnest in the eyelids. Its functions are: *sensation*, heat regulation, **absorption**, *protection*, *excretion* and *secretion* (which can be remembered by the acronym SHAPES).

Skin disorder – *skin dis-or-dur* – a **condition** of the skin that can occur as a result of an **infection**, the over-secretion of substances from the **glands** or an imbalance of a body function. For example, **folliculitis** is an infection of the **hair follicle** and is a **contraindication** to some hairdressing **services**.

Skin sensitivity – *skin sen-si-ti-vi-tee* – when an area of the skin or scalp may be tender or sore, which would be further aggravated by the carrying out of a **colouring service**. The **stylist** may be able to perform an 'off scalp' application, whereby the **product** can be applied using a **highlighting cap**, **foils** or mesh. See also **scalp irritation**.

Skin staining – *skin stay-ning* – marking of the skin caused by **barrier cream** not being applied, or the result of the poor application of a **colouring product**.

Skin tensioning – *skin ten-shun-ing* – stretching the skin taut during a **shaving service**, either behind or in front of the **razor** stroke, to provide a firm surface for the razor to glide over easily and quickly. Using the correct tension reduces the risk of cutting the client's skin.

Skin test – *skin test* – a test carried out before a **colouring service**, to check for any **allergic reactions** to the products that will be used on the client. A small dry area of skin just behind the ear is cleansed and a small mixture of the darkest colour, or the perm lotion, to be used on the client, mixed with 6% **hydrogen peroxide**, is applied to the area. This is left in place during the testing period. After 24 to 48 hours the patch is wiped clean from the skin with damp cotton wool. If the skin looks clear and is in the same condition as it was prior to testing the result is said to be a **negative reaction**. If the skin is raised, hot, red, with a rash, itchy, or if the eyes are puffy, this is known as a **positive** reaction and the proposed service cannot take place. Severe reactions include shortness of breath and may require medical attention. Also called **patch test** or **hypersensitivity test**.

Skin tone – *skin tow-n* – the colour of a client's skin, for example, a skin with an olive complexion.

Slices – *sliy-siz* – see **wraps**.

Slicing – *sliy-sing* – taking a section of hair from anywhere on the head and **colouring** it so that the colour stands out against the rest of the hair.

SMART targets – *smar-t tar-gitz* – an acronym (word formed from the initial letters of words) used in management to develop targets or goals (see **development targets**). The letters represent these words:

Specific: statements must be clear and plain

Measurable: goals and targets must be defined

Achievable: set only goals and targets that can be achieved

Realistic: objectives should be real rather than ideal

Time bound: there must be a start date and time and an end date and time.

Smoothing – *sm-oo-thing* – when **styling** hair, the outside layer of the hair is **blow-dried** so that the **cuticle** lies flat and smooth. The **airflow** from the **hairdryer** is directed so that it flows down the cuticle shaft from the roots to the points. This avoids lifting the cuticle and therefore making the hair appear fluffy and dull.

S/NVQ – *es-en-vee-kyoo* – stands for Scottish Vocational Qualification/**National Vocational Qualification**.

Sodium relaxer – *so-dee-um ree-lax-ur* – a **relaxing** product which, although is irritating to the scalp, is less drying on the hair. It penetrates through the cuticle quickly and leaves maximum shine. See also **non-sodium relaxer**.

Softening (stage) – *sof-ning* – one of the three stages of **perming** hair, when the **perm lotion** opens and swells the **cuticle** scales to allow the lotion to enter the **cortex**.

Spatula – *spat-u-lur* – a flat, wide-based **tool**, with teeth across the top edge, used to apply a **colouring product** to sections of hair. The hair is pulled through the tool to distribute colour evenly throughout the hair.

Special offer – *spesh-ul of-ur* – a short-term incentive or discount to encourage clients to invest in other **services** or try out new specialist **products**, for example, giving away a free **conditioner** with every perm.

Specialist treatment – *spesh-ul-ist treet-mnt* – a **treatment** which requires particular **training** and a higher level of skill to carry it out, for example, a **corrective relaxing** service or African Caribbean styling techniques.

Specified procedure – *spes-i-fiyd pru-see-jur* – a specific method used when carrying out a **service** such as **perming**, **colouring** or **relaxing**. It includes doing a **visual check** and performing any **necessary tests** on the hair beforehand.

Spiral curl – *spiy-rul kur-l* – a **curl** shaped in a spiral or ringlet. It can be achieved temporarily on longer hair using **curling tongs**.

Spiral perm winding – *spiy-rul purm-wiyn-ding* – an unconventional **perm winding** technique in which square sections of long hair are wound spirally up a **perm rod** to form long **spiral curls**. It creates little **root lift**.

Sprays – *spr-ay-z* – **hair spray** and **gel** spray, both **finishing products**, which give hold to the hair, add shine and give UV (ultra-violet) **protection** against the sun's rays. They also act as barriers to **atmospheric moisture**. Care must be taken not to use too much of these products as they can leave a white flaky residue on the hair. Both products are suitable for all hair types although gel spray is a heavier, wetter product so needs to be applied more sparingly on finer hair.

Square face shape – *sk-way-r fay-s shay-p* – the **head and face shape** determined by a broad forehead with an angular jaw line. The most suitable hairstyle for this shape should add a little height without width and taper well towards the jaw line to soften the squareness of the face. (See head and face shapes on page 161.)

Square neckline – *sk-way-r nek-liyn* – the shape determined by **cutting** a squared outline at the **nape** of the neck in which the corners of the hair **length** are left in place. Unwanted hair is removed from outside *continued...*

the neckline shape to produce a clean, accurate square result.

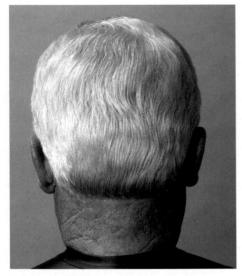

Square neckline

Stack perm winding – *stak purm wiyn-ding* – an unconventional *perm winding* technique. *Perm rods* are wound around sections of hair in the *nape* area first and subsequent rods are wound leaving more of the root and mid-length out as the hair is wound up the head. This creates a stacking effect and produces straight roots with curlier mid-lengths and ends.

Standardisation – *stan-dud-diy-zay-shun* – the way in which something conforms to a particular standard or quality, such as the *assessment* carried out on a candidate to gain an *S/NVQ qualification*.

Steamer – *steem-ur* – electrical equipment that produces moist heat to open the cuticle scales and aids penetration of conditioning products and bleaches. It helps with speeding up the developing of bleaching products as it does not dry out the product.

Sterilisation – *st-e-ril-iy-zay-shun* – the process of completely ridding material or tissue of live *micro-organisms*, leaving no viable forms of life. It is done by the use of:

- chemicals – using alcohol or **Barbicide®** (a disinfectant) to soak small *equipment*
- heat – putting towels and gowns into a boil wash cycle
- radiation – putting small equipment overnight in an ultra-violet (UV) ray box
- steam pressure – using an autoclave (apparatus which sterilises), for metallic equipment only.

See also *bacteria*, *infections* and *legislation*.

Stock – *st-ok* – all *products* used within a business. In a salon these include products for salon *services*, retail items, *equipment* used within the salon, consumables (disposable items), such as cotton wool and tissue, and semi-consumables (reusable items), such as aprons and gloves.

Stock control – *st-ok con-tr-ol* – the regulating and ordering of *stock*, by counting on a regular basis, to ensure good selling lines and most popular treatment lines are never sold out. See also *stock levels*.

Stock levels – *st-ok lev-ulz* – the amount of *stock* required to meet customer demands and allow *services* to continue. A minimum level is set (e.g. 14 of a popular *shampoo*) and the stock number should not fall below that. If it does, more is ordered, taking into account the time for the order to be delivered. This process ensures that items used regularly never run out.

Straighteners – *strayt-nurz* – electrical, heated *styling* *equipment* used for *smoothing* and *straightening* out movement present in the hair. Heat *protection* spray should be used during the process, as high levels of temperature are involved which, with prolonged use, will cause damage to the hair. Also called *straightening* irons.

Straightening – *strayt-ning* – a *styling* process that uses tension to pull out any *curl* or movement in the hair. Large round brushes are used as their compact bristles allow a firm grip to be used on the hair. During the *blow-drying* process, *hydrogen bonds* are broken down and re-formed to help the hair stay in its new position longer than if the hair is straightened using *straighteners* or a *pressing comb*.

Strand test – *stran-d-test* –

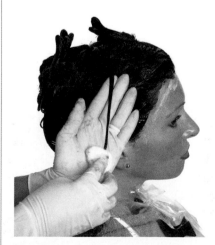

Strand test

continued...

135

a test to see how well a colour on the hair is processing or developing at intervals throughout a *colouring service*. A dampened piece of cotton wool is used to remove some of the excess tint to assess the colour.

Strop – *str-op* – a *tool* with canvas on one side and leather on the other, used to give the *razor* a smooth, clean and polished edge. Canvas on one side is used to clean the razor and leather on the other creates an effect similar to mild honing (see *hone*).

Styling – *s-tiy-ling* – a process of working with, and manipulating, the hair to change its shape, by moulding it around a *roller*, brush or piece of electrical *equipment*.

Styling aids – *s-tiy-ling ay-dz* – *styling* and *setting products* that help the *stylist* to manipulate the hair, and which give body, support and hold to the hair. Many contain conditioning agents and UV (ultra-violet) filters to protect and condition the client's hair. They also help to form a barrier on the hair, preventing *atmospheric moisture* from making the style collapse. See also *beta keratin* and *alpha keratin*.

Stylist – *s-tiy-list* – a fully trained, qualified hairdresser with a high level of *professional* skill and fully covered by *insurance*.

Subcutaneous layer – *sub-kyoo-tayn-ee-us lay-ur* – a layer of the skin, found beneath the *dermis* which contains fat cells and insulates against loss of heat. It also protects the internal organs of the body. (See the structure of the skin diagram on page 159.)

Subsection – *sub-sek-shun* – a *mesh of hair* taken after the hair is initially divided into sections. It is done so that the *stylist* can work in a methodical and logical way over the head.

Summary – *sum-ur-ee* – a brief account giving an overview of something.

Supplier – *sup-liy-ur* – a trader who sells materials, *equipment* and *products*, usually in bulk sizes or quantities.

Surface conditioner – *sur-fis kon-di-shun-ur* – a *conditioning product* that affects only the *cuticle* region of the hair. It closes the cuticle scales making the hair feel soft and look shiny. Types include cream rinses, anti-oxy conditioner and acid rinses, for example, lemon juice and vinegar.

Sweat – *sw-et* – liquid that is excreted onto the skin to cool body temperature and remove waste products.

Sweat glands – *sw-et gl-and-z* – *glands* found in the *dermis* of the skin and which open onto the skin's surface. They produce *sweat* which is a mixture of salt, water and waste products. Sweat helps to cool the body temperature as it evaporates (disappears) on the skin's surface. When combined with *sebum* it

helps form the *acid mantle* to protect the skin. (See the structure of the skin diagram on page 159.)

SWOT analysis – *sw-ot un-al-i-sis* – an *analysis* of a business to examine its **s**trengths, **w**eaknesses, **o**pportunities and **t**hreats.

Synthetic fibre extensions – *sin-thet-ik f-iy-bur ex-ten-shunz* – man-made *hair extensions* which come in a large range of colours, including vibrant colours for an unconventional or extreme look. They are generally cheaper to use than human hair extensions, but are not as easy to maintain. See also *added hair*.

Takings – *tay-kings* – the amount of money earned by a business.

Tangle – *tang-l* – to intertwine in a confused mass. When dividing and separating hair extensions it is important not to tangle the hair.

Tapered cut – *tay-purd kut* – a haircut which has soft outlines that fade, leaving no harsh lines and following the natural shape of the hairline. See also *tapering*.

Tapered neckline – *tay-purd nek-liyn* – the shape determined by a soft, faded outline, without leaving harsh lines, which follows the natural shape of the hairline around the neck. It is achieved by cutting the hair very short into the *nape* area, either using **clipper-over-comb** or **scissor-over-comb** techniques or **clippers**. Unwanted hair is removed from outside the neckline shape to produce a clean, accurate, tapered result.

Tapering – *tay-pur-ing* – a **cutting** technique whereby the blades of the scissors are opened and closed slightly while sliding the scissors up and down the hair shaft (using a flicking of the wrist action).

Tapotement – *tap-ote-mnt* – one of five types of massage movements used over the scalp. This is an invigorating motion, using the pads of the fingers in a firm tapping rhythm. It stimulates the scalp, increases blood flow to the scalp and **hair follicles**, and releases muscular tension. See also **effleurage massage**, **petrissage massage**, **friction massage**, **rotary massage**.

Target – *tar-git* – a realistic **objective** or goal to be achieved, usually within a set time scale (see **SMART**). There may be incentives or rewards to be won which can

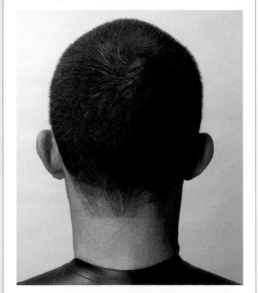

Tapered neckline

be personal – to provide motivation within a *job role* – or general: for the whole salon to take part in, for example, *selling* all particular hair products in *stock*. See also *development targets*.

Target colour – *tar-git kul-ur* – the final colour a hairdresser is aiming for in a *colouring service*, based on the client's choice.

Target group – *tar-git groo-p* – a specific group of people for whom a product or event is aimed towards. See also *promotions*.

Task – *tar-sk* – a job or specific *responsibility*.

Team members – *teem mem-burz* – a group of people who work together as one unit.

Teasing – *tee-zing* – a technique which adds gentle lift and support to the hair. It is done using a *dressing-out comb*, by gently pushing back into the hair to lightly matt the root area. This technique is good for adding light support and taking out roller marks that may have be left from a *setting* process.

Telogen – *tel-u-jen* – a stage at the end of the *hair growth cycle*. It is the resting stage of hair growth, when the *hair follicle* is waiting to start growing again. It lasts between three and four months and at the end of this phase, the follicle re-enters the *anagen* phase and the *papilla* becomes active again, ready for the growth of a new hair. During this time the hair does not receive any nourishment from the blood supply and so it eventually falls out. Approximately 50 to 100 hairs a day are lost, but are normally replaced with new ones entering from the anagen phase. *Baldness* occurs when the telogen stage lasts indefinitely and the anagen phase of the follicle does not start. (See the hair growth cycle diagram on page 160.)

Temperature – *tem-pru-chur* – a measure of how hot or cold something is. An increase or decrease in temperature is a factor to consider when performing a hairdressing *service*. For example, during a *colouring service* the room temperature, and the amount of body heat (heat given off by the body) that is released, will affect the timings and processing of the colour; the hotter the room the *continued...*

quicker the development of the colour. A very cold room will slow down the development of the colour.

Temporary colour – *tem-por-ur-ee kul-ur* – a product that comes in the form of *mousse*, *sprays*, *gels* and hair mascara (colour that is applied using a wand) and temporarily colours hair. It can darken the hair or change its tone and is removed from the hair completely on the first *shampoo*. It does not have the ability to lighten hair colour.

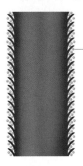

Colour particles on the cuticle and outside the hair shaft only.

Effect of temporary colour on hair structure

Tender – *ten-dur* – a term for money and non-cash payments considered acceptable for payment of goods or services. See also *legal tender*.

Tension – *ten-shun* – how firmly a *mesh of hair* is held during a hairdressing *service*. It should always be even for all services, as uneven tension will produce, for example, an uneven curl in *rollering* or *perming*, or, in cutting, an unbalanced look.

Terminal hair – *tur-min-ul hayr* – see *hair types*.

Test cutting – *test kut-ing* – a small cutting of a client's hair taken to test the suitability of *colouring products* on the hair and to check that the desired colour will be achieved. A few strands are taken from the part of the head to be treated and secured together with tape to keep it all together. The hair strand is then placed in a non-metallic bowl. A small amount of the required colour/s is mixed with the correct strength of *hydrogen peroxide* and added to the hair, coating it well, just as it would be done on the head. The *manufacturer's instructions* for processing time are followed and the hair is rinsed and dried to see the results. The outcome is discussed with the client to determine whether or not to proceed with the colouring service.

Test result – *test ruz-ult* – the outcome of a test, usually performed before a hairdressing *service* is carried out. It shows the strength and *condition* of the hair and whether there are any *products* that will react with the hair during the service. See also *necessary tests*, *allergic reaction*, *negative reactions*.

Tetanus – *tet-n-us* – a bacterial *infection* which causes violent muscle spasms. A tetanus jab is given every ten years and after a suspect injury such as a cut from a rusty blade. Hairdressers commonly nip their skin with scissors, so they should ensure that their *immunisation* against the *disease* is up to date.

Texture test – *tex-chur test* – see *porosity test*.

Texturising – *tex-chur-iy-zing* – removing weight or bulk from a hairstyle to enhance and personalise it. It is a type of *thinning*. Sometimes called weave cutting, pointing/chipping in, castle cutting, *razoring*.

Texturising scissors – *tex-chur-iy-zing siz-urz* – see *thinning scissors*.

Theme – *th-eem* – a central topic, basis or idea, for example,

using *avant-garde* styles in a *hair show*.

Thermal heating stove – *thur-mul hee-ting sto-v* – *equipment* used to heat non-electrical *pressing combs* and *curling tongs* when *thermal styling*, for example, to temporarily straighten or curl hair.

Thermal styling – *thur-mul stiy-ling* – physically straightening or curling hair temporarily using a physical process. See also *thermal styling tools*.

Thermal styling tools – *thur-mul stiy-ling tool-z* – tools used when *thermal styling*, such as a *pressing comb* and *curling tongs*.

Thinning – *thin-ing* – reducing the bulk within a *hairstyle* using *cutting* techniques such as *razoring* or *texturising*. See also *thinning scissors*.

Thinning scissors – *thin-ing siz-urz* – scissors with *serrated* edges, used to remove bulk from the hair. Scissors with only one serrated blade remove less bulk from the hair; if both blades are serrated, then more bulk *continued...*

141

can be removed. If the degree of serration is increased, a much more textured look can be achieved. Also known as *texturising scissors*, *serrated scissors*, *notched scissors*.

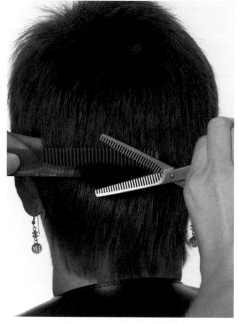

Thinning scissors

Time management – *tiym man-ij-mnt* – the practice of using one's time sensibly and wisely. Making lists and working through them, allotting a time to each task and being organised help to manage time in a *productive* way.

Timescale – *tiym-skay-l* – an allotted amount of time allowed, or given, to work on and finish a task.

Tinea – *tin-ee-ur* – see *ringworm*.

Tinting bowl – *tin-ting bo-l* – a plastic bowl with measurement markings used to measure and mix *colouring products*. Also called **tint bowl**.

Tinting brush – *tin-ting br-ush* – a plastic brush with bristles used to apply *colouring products* to the hair. It can vary in size and shape, according to the current or emerging styles being performed in a salon, or be used alongside new products that come onto the market which require a specific tool. Also called **tint brush**.

Tone – *tow-n* – the colour that can be seen in hair, for example, copper, red, mahogany.

Tool – *too-l* – a piece of *equipment* used to perform a *service* and which is usually held in the hands, such as *scissors*, *rollers* and so on.

Toxicity – *tox-is-it-ee* – the degree of poison contained within a substance which is harmful to health.

Traction alopecia – *trak-shun al-o-pee-sha* – hair thinning or loss due to **excessive tension** on the **hair follicle**. This can be as a result of wearing the hair in tight **braids** or **plaits**. The source of the tension needs to be removed and the client may need to be **referred** to a **trichologist**.

Trade Descriptions Act 1968 and 1972 – *tray-d dus-krip-shunz akt* – this Act concerns the selling of products. A business:

- cannot give false or misleading information about products
- must ensure labels on products are displayed clearly.

Trading periods – *tray-ding peer-yuds* – set times in a day when a business is open. For a salon, the busiest times are usually Saturdays and late night openings.

Training – *tray-ning* – the education, **guidance** or **instruction** of new skills and techniques, **product** use or product knowledge, given to keep staff up to date with current trends and emerging client demands. It can be done in the salon or at an external venue; product companies offer training when a salon has purchased equipment or products. See also **continuing professional development**, **development targets**.

Treatments – *treet-mnts* – the range of **services** available to a client within a salon.

Treatment conditioners – *treet-mnt kon-di-shun-urz* – **products** used to condition or improve the health of the hair and scalp. They are specially formulated with ingredients to improve a specific problem, such as regulating over-active **sebaceous glands** or decreasing the production of **epidermal** cells.

Treatment knowledge – *treet-mnt no-lij* – knowledge about all the **services** on offer in a salon. An employee should have the ability to explain them to a client, even if he or she cannot perform them.

Treatment shampoo – *treet-mnt sham-poo* – a **shampoo** used not only to cleanse *continued...*

but also to improve the health of the hair and scalp.

Triangular face shape – *triy-ang-yoo-lur fay-s shay-p* – a *head and face shape*, similar to a heart face shape, but not as soft in outline. The ideal hairstyle should aim to reduce the width of the jawline, by emphasising the forehead. The hair should be worn close at the cheekbones with fullness in the jawline area.

Trichologist – *tri-kol-o-jist* – a person who has studied *trichology* and is qualified to diagnose (identify) and treat scalp and hair *diseases* and *disorders*. In the United Kingdom, The Institute of Trichologists publishes a Code of Professional Practice and Ethics, by which all practising trichologists who are registered members of the Institute are expected to abide. See also **Code of Practice**.

Trichology – *tri-kol-o-jee* – the science and study of the structure, function and *diseases* of the human hair and scalp. The clinical branch deals with the diagnosis (identification) and treatment of diseases and *disorders* of human hair and scalp.

Twist – *tw-ist* – (also known as *Bantu knot*) hair shaped in a spiral, achieved by *twisting* each section of hair on itself. How tight, loose, large or small it will be depends on the size of the section taken.

Twisting – *tw-ist-ing* – (also known as **comb twist**) a dressing technique used for *styling* medium to longer length hair. A *pintail comb* is used to take a section of hair from the front hairline. Starting at the roots, the hair is turned in the same direction down to the points of the hair until the desired *twist* is achieved.

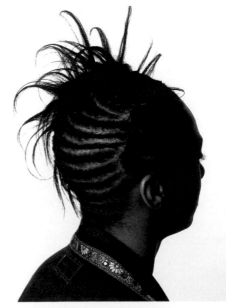

Hairstyle using twisting techniques

Two-strand twist – *too-str-and tw-ist* – two-strand twists are similar to braiding except two strands of hair are twisted together instead of three.

T-zone – *tee-zown* – a section of hair from just below the crown to the forehead, and extending from ear to ear, shaped like a 'T' if looked at from above. Also called **T-bar**.

Under-processing – *un-dur pro-ses-ing* – when a **chemical service** has not reached its full development time and does not produce the results expected.

Uneven result – *un-ee-vn ru-zul-t* – when the required result of a **chemical service** is not consistent over the whole head. For example, the formation of irregular **curl** or a patchy result from **colouring**, due to using incorrect techniques, not taking into account **hot spots** or testing the **porosity of hair** beforehand.

Unfair Contract Terms Act 1977 / Unfair Terms in Consumer Contracts Regulations 1999 – *un-fayr kon-trakt turmz akt / un-fayr turmz in kon-syoo-mur kon-trakts reg-yoo-lay-shunz* – these two Acts allow a client to challenge any terms of a contract they have signed with a salon, if it is unfair or unreasonable.

Uniform curl – *yoo-ni-form kur-l* – correct and even amount of **curl** achieved along the whole **length** of the hair.

Uniform layer – *yoo-ni-form lay-ur* – when the internal and external sections of the hair are of the same length. This is done by holding the hair and cutting it at a 90 degree angle from the head.

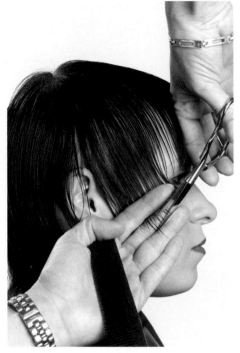

Ensuring a uniform, even shape

Unit – *yoo-nit* – the grouping of a particular set of skills for a subject of which a candidate needs to gain competency. Each is made up of several **elements** and the completion of a unit will be awarded by an **assessor** only after it has been fully achieved. It is possible to gain units of credit and partial certification if a candidate has completed lots of units, but not the full **qualification**. Units usually stay active for about three years and a candidate can return to the **assessment centre** to make up a full qualification within that time, without having to retake any of them. See also **mandatory units**, **optional units**.

Unravel – *un-ra-v-l* – to untangle or untwist. For example, clients are encouraged to return to the salon six to eight weeks after a **locking** service to re-twist the **locks** to ensure this does not happen. If synthetic hair is used, the ends can be burnt to fuse them together to prevent unravelling.

Value – *val-yoo* – 1. the cost of something, which reflects its worth. 2. to realise the importance of someone or something, such as a regular salon client.

Velcro rollers – *vel-kro ro-lurz* – rigid plastic cylinders used to curl hair. Small holes on their surface allow heat to penetrate through them to aid the drying process. Covered with a looped felt layer used to attach each roller to the hair, they are used for *dry setting* services in conjunction with *styling* products to support the *curl*.

Vellus hair – *vel-us hayr* – see *hair types*.

Venue – *ven-yoo* – a place where an exhibition, show or demonstration takes place that is open to the public to view, such as a hall or function suite in a hotel. When organising a hairdressing event it is essential that the venue is large enough for the purpose and its facilities comply with *health and safety*. See also *hair show*, *competition work*.

Vertical roll – *vur-ti-kul ro-l* – a dressing technique for long hair in which the hair is styled into a roll at the centre back of the head running from the *nape* (the narrowest section of the roll) to the *crown* (the widest section of the roll). This type of roll can be secured anywhere on the head, depending on the desired effect. Also called *French pleat*.

Vibrate – *viy-bray-t* – to make fine, trembling movements to and fro, for example, when applying some massage movements. Pressure is applied using either the fingertips or the palms of the hands against the scalp; this clears nerve pathways and relieves tension in the muscles.

Vibro-massage – *viy-bro-mas-arj* – a massage technique carried out using a mechanical, hand-held massage device which *vibrates*. It stimulates blood flow to the skin and production of *sebum* from the *sebaceous glands* and helps to relax muscles and improve muscle tone.

Virgin hair – *vur-jin hayr* – hair that has not been chemically treated.

Virus – *viy-rus* – (plural **viruses** – *viy-rus-ez*) – an *infection*-producing agent, only visible through an electron microscope, which multiplies within living cells. Viruses can gain entry into the body through the lungs in airborne droplets, through eating, a break or cut in the skin, or through a blood transfusion. Some viral diseases are chickenpox, the common cold, influenza (flu), rabies, polio, herpes (cold sores), yellow fever and mumps.

Visual aid – *viz-yool ayd* – a picture or an illustration used to show an example of something. For example, a hairdresser may show a client a picture of an intended look from a *styling* magazine, or a colour on the colour chart.

Visual check – *viz-yool chek* – to view something to gain information about its *condition*, for example, looking and checking the scalp and hair, prior to a *service*, to determine if there are any *contraindications* to the requested service being carried out – some skin or hair *disorders*, *diseases* and *infestations*, such as *ringworm* or *head lice*, need a *medical referral*. It also allows the hairdresser to recognise a condition which may require

specialist *treatment*, such as severe *dandruff*, or the use of specific *products*. The final *hairstyle* is always checked for *balance* in shape, style and *length* to ensure that the overall result is correct.

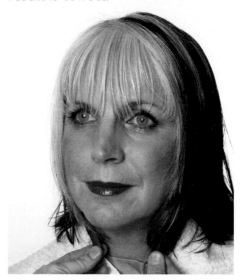
Checking evenness in length

Volume – *vol-yoo-m* – the fullness or thickness of hair.

Voucher – *vow-chur* – a non-cash payment slip, usually with an amount printed on it, treated as equal in *value* to the same amount of *cash* in the salon till. See also *cash equivalent*.

Warm tones – *wor-m tow-nz* – colours that contain yellow, orange, copper, red, brunette or mahogany.

Water spray – *wor-tur sp-ray* – a spray bottle filled with water, used to wet hair during *services* such as *cutting* to ensure consistency throughout the cut. If the hair is left to dry out during the cut the hair *lengths* may become uneven.

Water temperature – *wor-tur tem-pru-chur* – the degree of heat in water. It is important to test this, especially before shampooing a client's hair.

Waving – *way-ving* – the physical process of using heated *styling equipment* to add a temporary wave (a slight curl) to the hair.

Wax – *wax* – a *finishing product* used at the end of a *styling* process to define and add texture to the finished *hairstyle*. A small amount only is placed in the palm and massaged evenly into the hands before gently distributing it on the client's hair. It is not suitable for very fine hair

as it will be too heavy and weigh the hair down.

Weave perm winding – *wee-v purm wiyn-ding* – an unconventional *perm winding* technique in which sections of hair are wound onto *perm rods* in any direction while other sections of hair are left unwound. Care must be taken to ensure *perm lotion* and *neutraliser* do not touch the weaved-out sections. Different textures throughout the hair are achieved with this technique.

Weaving – *wee-ving* – a technique in which parts of the hair, rather than the whole head, are coloured (see *highlighting* and *lowlighting*). A section of hair is taken and the end of a *pintail comb* is dipped in and out of it to remove pieces of hair. These *meshes of hair* are held in place and coloured, while the untouched hair is left either as natural colour or filled in with a different colour. This technique is used so the *stylist* can place the colour exactly where it is needed.

Weight – *wayt* – the amount of bulk within a hairstyle.

Wet setting – *wet set-ing* – a *setting* method whereby the hair is shampooed before applying *setting aids*. This breaks down the *hydrogen bonds* in the hair which allows the shape of the hair to be changed. See also *dry setting*.

Wet setting rollers – *wet set-ing ro-lurz* – rigid plastic cylinders, with small holes, used to curl hair in a *wet setting* process. A section of hair is wound around each one and a pin is passed through the holes to secure the roller to the hair. The holes on the surface allow heat from the hood dryer/hairdryer to penetrate the roller, and as the hair is dried in this position, it takes on the shape of the roller.

White hair – *wiy-t hayr* – hair which does not contain any colour *pigment*. The *percentage of white hair* on a client will influence the type of colour and choice of *hydrogen peroxide* used during a *colouring* service.

White light – *wiy-t liyt* – natural daylight, such as sunlight at noon. It is the best type of light for looking closely at the hair colour as the *tones* are not affected in the way they are with artificial lighting. For example, tungsten lighting gives off a yellow hue, making colours look warmer and neutralising ash tones in the hair; fluorescent lighting gives off a blue hue, making ash colours appear more ash and neutralising warm tones in the hair.

Whooping cough – *hoop-ing kof* – a *disease* caused by a bacterial *infection* which causes a spasm of coughing, followed by a particular sound – hence its name. This *contagious* disease is seen mainly in children who have not been *immunised* against the disease.

Widow's peak – *wid-owz pee-k* – a *hair growth pattern* in which the hairline at the front of the forehead grows downwards at the centre, forming a 'V' shape of hair and two half circles of hair either side of it. Cutting a *fringe* is difficult, especially with fine hair, as the hair will lift up and separate into the V shape. It is best to work with the natural hair growth to *complement* the face and hair texture.

Wind – *wiynd* – to twist the hair in a circular direction, often around itself. See also *brick perm winding*, *directional* continued...

151

winding, *double perm winding*, *hopscotch perm winding*, *nine section perm winding*, *root perm winding*, *root to point winding*, *spiral perm winding*, *stack perm winding*, *weave perm winding*.

Winding technique – *wiyn-ding tek-neek* – a method used to *wind* hair. See also *perm winding*.

With a fringe – *with u frinj* – a phrase applied to a *hairstyle* which incorporates a visible *fringe*.

With a parting – *with u par-ting* – a phrase applied to a *hairstyle* which incorporates a visible *parting*.

With ears exposed – *with ee-yrz ex-po-zd* – a phrase applied to a *hairstyle* which allows the ears to be seen.

Without a fringe – *with-owt u frinj* – a phrase applied to a *hairstyle* which does not incorporate a visible *fringe*.

Without a parting – *with-owt u par-ting* – a phrase applied to a *hairstyle* which does not incorporate a visible *parting*.

Witness statement – *wit-nis stay-t-mnt* – a signed and dated testimony of an account of events observed by a person. It is one form of **evidence** that can be added to an **S/NVQ** candidate's **portfolio**, and can be given by a line manager, a client, or a colleague, but not an **assessor**.

Workforce development – *wurk-for-s duv-el-up-mnt* – activities which increase the ability of **S/NVQ** candidates to participate effectively in the **workplace**. It includes industry **training** days and certificates gained in a salon, outside of college or the **assessment** centre, for example, a first-aid **qualification**.

Working practices – *wurk-ing prak-tis-ez* – standard practices that all staff must follow. In a salon, they include the correct use of materials, **treatment** procedures and working techniques used whilst offering a hairdressing **service** to clients.

Working Time Directive 1998 – *wurk-ing tiym diy-rek-tiv* – the aim of this directive is to prevent employees working excessive hours. It stipulates that employers:

- must not allow employees to work more than 48 hours a week (unless an employee wishes to do so)
- must allow employees a rest period of 11 hours between each working day, and 24 hours rest in each 7 day period
- must allow an employee to take a 20 minute break after 6 consecutive hours of work
- must allow a minimum of 4 paid weeks holiday a year for full-time workers, and a pro-rata entitlement for part-time and casual workers.

Workplace – *wurk play-s* – the place in which a person works. In a salon, it includes the area where hairdressing *services* take place and places where practical services are not carried out, such as the *reception*, *consultation* rooms and the washrooms. *Health and safety* standards apply to every section in the workplace.

Workplace (Health, Safety and Welfare) Regulations 1992 – *wurk-play-s hel-th sayf-tee nd wel-fayr reg-yoo-lay-shunz* – these regulations stipulate that employers must provide a proper and safe working environment for their employees. They must: maintain all equipment and systems in use, ensure reasonable working temperatures, provide sufficient lighting, keep the premises clean and tidy, provide suitable washing and toilet facilities. Changing of clothing, catering provisions, safe disposal of waste materials, along with clean drinking water also need to be provided.

Workplace policies/procedures – *wurk-play-s pol-i-seez / pru-see-jurz* – directives put in place to ensure staff are aware of the correct *procedures* and *policies* that must be adhered to in a *workplace*. They include general and salon specific *health and safety* practices, *personal conduct* for staff, *pricing structures* for treatments and *customer services* information.

Work product – *wurk pro-duk-t* – a term applied to the result of an *S/NVQ* candidate's work, such as a completed record, a *health and safety* book, or the preparation of a piece of equipment ready for use. It should be shown to, and discussed with, the candidate's *assessor* before being documented.

153

Woven effects – *wo-vn u-fek-ts* – a dressing technique for **styling** long hair. Strands of hair are **intertwined** to produce a style resembling a woven basket.

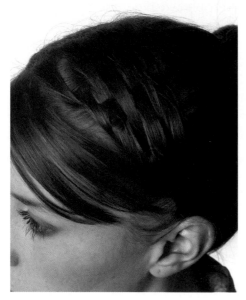

Woven effects

Wrapping – *rap-ing* – the technique of adding hair, yarn, wool or silk by wrapping it around a **lock** of hair resulting in an overall compact look to the hair (see **yarn locks**). The length of yarn is held a quarter of the way down the client's hair, then, while holding a section of hair securely, the yarn is wrapped around the hair, starting from the roots and working down the length of the hair by twisting it in a spiral fashion. The term also applies to hair being wrapped in a silk or satin scarf at night to prevent hair becoming frizzy and dry.

Wraps – *rap-s* – flat sheets of a foam-type substance, easy to tear and fold, which stick to the **colouring product** during a colouring **service**. They can be moulded to the shape of the head. They are used to cover **block colour** sections and prevent the dye coming into contact with areas of hair that are not to be coloured. Also called **slices**.

Written questions – *rit-tn kwes-chunz* – formal and informal (e.g. multiple-choice) **questions** given by a tutor or an **assessor** to an **S/NVQ** candidate to complete. The answers to these can be written or typed, or given orally. They are useful for revision to see how much a candidate has retained.

Yarn locks – *yar-n lox* – *locks* created using a variety of yarn and wool fibres. The wool or yarn is plaited into the hair to create a *dreadlocks* effect and is used when a client does not want to wait for his or her hair to grow and begin to lock. It is important to continually detangle the hair and avoid pulling, dragging and overloading the hair with products. If the hair is left *wrapped* for a minimum of three to four months it should result in natural hair locking. The locks can be used as a foundation to produce mature ones.

Appendix

The structure of the skin

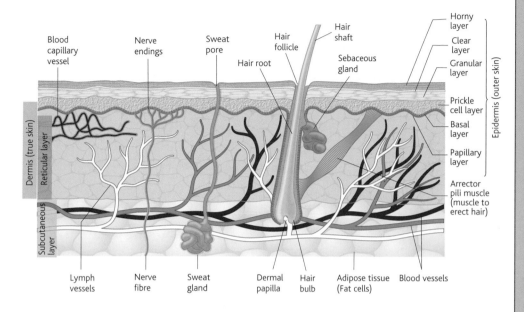

Blood capillary vessel

Nerve endings

Sweat pore

Hair follicle

Hair shaft

Hair root

Sebaceous gland

Horny layer

Clear layer

Granular layer

Prickle cell layer

Basal layer

Papillary layer

Arrector pili muscle (muscle to erect hair)

Dermis (true skin)

Reticular layer

Subcutaneous layer

Epidermis (outer skin)

Lymph vessels

Nerve fibre

Sweat gland

Dermal papilla

Hair bulb

Adipose tissue (Fat cells)

Blood vessels

The hair follicle

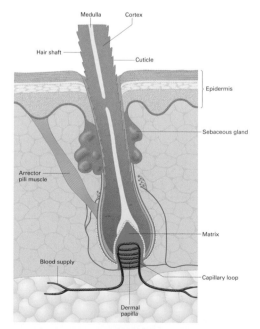

Medulla

Cortex

Hair shaft

Cuticle

Epidermis

Sebaceous gland

Arrector pili muscle

Matrix

Blood supply

Capillary loop

Dermal papilla

A vertical cross-section of a hair in its follicle

Appendix

The hair growth cycle

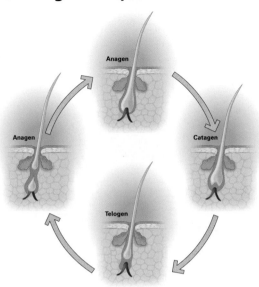

The cortex

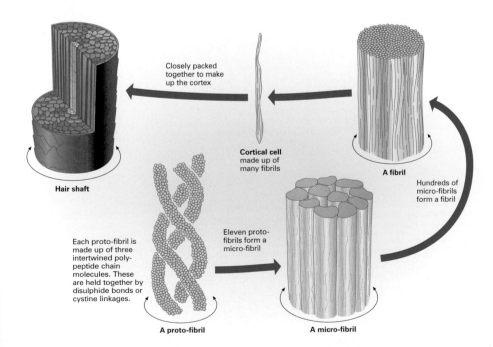

Closely packed together to make up the cortex

Cortical cell made up of many fibrils

A fibril

Hundreds of micro-fibrils form a fibril

Hair shaft

Each proto-fibril is made up of three intertwined poly-peptide chain molecules. These are held together by disulphide bonds or cystine linkages.

Eleven proto-fibrils form a micro-fibril

A proto-fibril

A micro-fibril

Head and face shapes

Oval

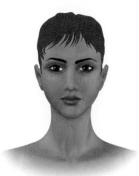

Round

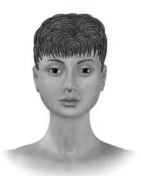

Square

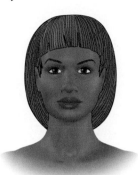

Oblong

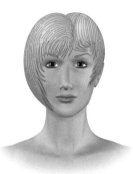

Heart shaped

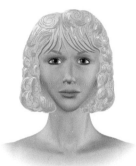

Diamond shaped

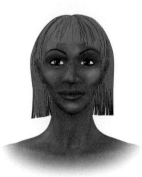

Pear shaped

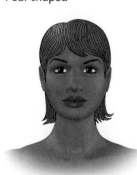

Triangular shaped

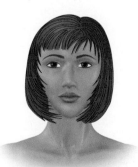

Common infectious diseases of the skin and scalp

Name	Recognised by
Scabies 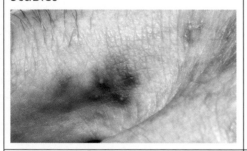	*Symptoms*: A rash of red, raised spots and severe itching, especially at night. *Refer to*: GP
Head lice 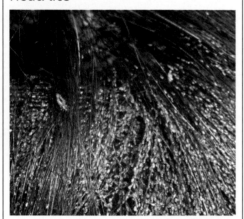	*Symptoms*: Intense itching, white or light brown specks which indicates the presence of nits (small eggs attached to the hair shaft close to the scalp, often at the nape of the neck and behind the ears). Lice may be present. Common in children. *Refer to*: Pharmacist or GP
Ringworm 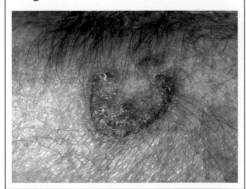	*Symptoms*: Red spot which enlarges and forms a ring with a raised red, scaly border. Contains broken hairs which may become brittle and fall out leaving bald patches. *Refer to*: GP

Name	Recognised by
Impetigo 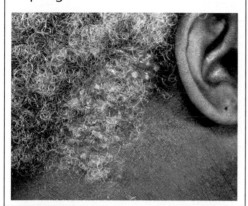	*Symptoms*: Small blisters, most commonly seen on the face, containing pus that may break and form a yellow crust. *Refer to*: GP
Folliculitis 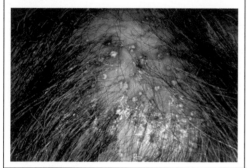	*Symptoms*: Small yellow pustules with hair in centre. *Refer to*: GP
Barber's itch (Sycosis barbae) 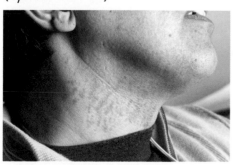	*Symptoms*: A form of folliculitis. Small red spots often with a yellow pustule around the follicle opening. General irritation and inflammation, with possible burning sensation. Found in the beard area. *Refer to*: GP

A summary of relevant legislation

Legislation is the process of making laws for the protection of all in society and business. You will encounter a lot of legislation in the study and industry of hairdressing and barbering.

Consumer Protection Act 1987

Consumer Safety Act 1978

Control of Substances Hazardous to Health Regulations 2002 (COSHH)

Cosmetic Products (Safety) Regulations 2004

Data Protection Act 1998

Disability Discrimination Act 1992, 1995 and 2005

Electricity at Work Regulations 1989

Employers' Liability (Compulsory Insurance) Act 1969

Fire Precautions (Workplace) Regulations 1997

General Product Safety Regulations 1994

Health and Safety at Work Act 1974 (HASAWA)

Manual Handling Operations Regulations 1992

Personal Protective Equipment at Work Regulations 1992 (PPE)

Prices Act 1974

Provision and Use of Work Equipment Regulations 1998

Race Relations Act 1976 (amended 2000)

Reporting of Injuries, Diseases and Dangerous Occurrences Regulations 1995 (RIDDOR)

Resale Prices Act 1964 and 1976

Sale of Goods Act 1979

Sale and Supply of Goods Act 1994

Sex Discrimination Act 1975 and 1986

Supply of Goods and Services Act 1982

Supply of Goods to Consumers Act 1994

Trade Descriptions Act 1968 and 1972

Unfair Contract Terms Act 1977/Unfair Terms in Consumer Contracts Regulations 1999

Workplace (Health, Safety and Welfare) Regulations 1992

Working Time Directive 1998

Related items

Code of Practice

Insurance

- Professional Indemnity Insurance
- Public Liability Insurance

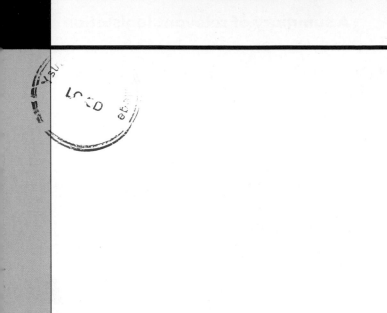